More praise for
The Magnesium Miracle

"Every doctor and patient should read this comprehensive book on the many roles of magnesium. . . . I loved this book. Clearly written and packed with information, it offers a compendium on natural medicine and is an invaluable resource for both practitioner and public alike. It is the most comprehensive and well-referenced guide to the myriad benefits of magnesium published to date."

—CAROLYN DEMARCO, M.D.,
author of *Take Charge of Your Body:
Women's Health Advisor*

"Throughout this volume and with utmost clarity, Carolyn Dean presents invaluable recommendations—based on the latest magnesium research. Virtually every American can benefit."

—PAUL PITCHFORD,
author of *Healing with Whole Foods:
Asian Traditions and Modern Nutrition*

"Physicians and therapists have paid scant attention to this very important element, which is also involved in maintaining our good health. The massive evidence is here in this important book on magnesium. I am pleased to have been taking magnesium for so many years."

—ABRAM HOFFER, M.D.,
author of *Putting It All Together:
The New Orthomolecular Nutrition*

"Excellent research together with valuable inspiration to empower the doctor within each of us."

—JOSHUA ROSENTHAL,
director of the Institute
for Integrative Nutrition,
author of *The Energy Balance Diet*

"An enlightening and practical book. Dr. Dean supplies powerful information for people while trumpeting a reminder to doctors about this essential and often overlooked mineral elixir. *The Magnesium Miracle* should be required reading for living a rich, healthy life."

—EUGENE CHARLES, D.C., DIBAK,
author of *Physician Heal Thy Patient*
and *Becoming Healthy, Wealthy and Wise*

"I have been in complementary medicine for thirty years and I believed I knew all there was to know about magnesium—until I [read] the latest book by Dr. Carolyn Dean. This book is the most comprehensive review on the subject I have ever read. As one can expect from a physician with such vast and diversified knowledge, *The Magnesium Miracle* contains information on allied fields of medicine that makes this book an incredible resource for doctors and patients alike. *The Magnesium Miracle* is a book that is going to be of great service to humanity since, as the author points out, there is so much information on magnesium that has failed to be included in the medical curriculum."

—SERAFINA CORSELLO, M.D.,
Wellness Medical Center for Integrative
Medicine, author of *Ageless Healing*

THE
MAGNESIUM
MIRACLE

THE MAGNESIUM MIRACLE

(Originally published as
The Miracle of Magnesium)

Carolyn Dean, M.D., N.D.

Ballantine Books New York

To the Miracle Women in my life:

my mum, Rena; my three sisters, Chris (who

labored with me on the first drafts of "the wee maggie"),

Anne, and Evelyn; and my agent, Beth.

Thank you all.

"Clearly there is more to life than magnesium" is one of the remarks from Dr. Dean's remarkable, almost encyclopedic, but very readable book. Her book is long overdue, for it gives the lay reader a chance to discover for him- or herself the many needs for this mineral in a healthy diet, and the reasons why this has not been emphasized in the everyday literature.

The requirement for magnesium in our diet is indeed a much neglected topic, and this book by Dr. Dean brings the message home by her carefully written repetitive emphasis on the subject. That does not mean that there are not many other nutrients necessary in our daily food intake, as stated above, but the point she so clearly makes is that the public in general has not been notified to look for the proper amount of this mineral in the daily diet and of the many reasons magnesium is needed in our bodies.

After a cursory overview of the material, the book should be read as one would read an encyclopedia, that is, pick out the parts one is particularly interested in, and then go back and try to read it all. This way the reader will get the gist of how important magnesium really is and how little he or she has been informed, be it from newspapers, magazines, or the rest of the news media. As the old adage says, "An ounce of prevention is worth a pound of cure," and so it is with balanced nutrition, which includes this all-important mineral in adequate amounts. (As to the other interesting parts of the book, our qualifications allow us to comment only on the material pertaining to the scientific basis for the need of magnesium.)

DR. BELLA T. ALTURA
Research Professor of Physiology and Pharmacology
SUNY Downstate Medical Center
Brooklyn, New York

DR. BURTON M. ALTURA
Professor of Physiology, Pharmacology, and Medicine
SUNY Downstate Medical Center
Brooklyn, New York

CONTENTS

PART THREE: THE RESEARCH CONTINUES

PART FOUR: TESTING AND SUPPLEMENTS

AUTHOR'S NOTE TO
THE REVISED EDITION

It is gratifying to know that since the first edition of *The Magnesium Miracle* was published in 2003, thousands of people have benefited from increasing the magnesium in their lives. Many people from around the world have sought me out through my Web site at www.carolyndean.com to share their magnesium success stories and for nutritional and wellness consultations with me by phone.

Many of the miraculous magnesium stories that I hear involve heart symptoms, severe cramping, PMS, anxiety, and depression. One woman rushed her husband to the hospital with chest pain, sweating, and shortness of breath—all the symptoms of a heart attack. After two days and many tests, the doctors could find nothing abnormal and released him. During her own research, this woman found the first edition of *The Magnesium Miracle* and realized her husband's chest pain might well be due to coronary artery spasms. She told his doctor about her research, and he agreed that magnesium should be tried. The miraculous result was that her husband had no more chest pain. Seeing her own symptoms in the pages of *The*

Magnesium Miracle, she took magnesium to reverse her moody PMS.

Most people with chronic fatigue syndrome and fibromyalgia improve about 50 percent when they begin to use magnesium. People who take magnesium for muscle spasms have shared that their mild depression and irritability disappear as a wonderful side benefit. One benefit of magnesium, which is difficult to prove scientifically, is a greater enjoyment of sexual activity, reported by many women. I've written about magnesium oil in this edition of *The Magnesium Miracle*, but already my clients are remarking on its many benefits. You can rub it into the gums to help treat inflammation and prevent bad breath and gum bleeding. Applied as a spray, it makes the skin smooth and soft.

Invariably, people who take magnesium for one symptom find that it improves many others, and they immediately begin telling their family and friends about it. One woman said that she has given away fifteen books; another gentleman ordered a case to give out to friends. This word-of-mouth spread of information about magnesium is truly improving health and changing lives.

Magnesium education received a boost in March 2005 when the George and Patsy Eby Foundation provided a grant that purchased 1,000 books each of *The Magnesium Miracle* and *The Magnesium Factor* by Mildred Seelig, M.D., and Andrea Rosanoff, Ph.D., to be given to members of Congress. Dr. Rosanoff and I hosted a reception on Capitol Hill to which members of Congress and their staff were invited and presented with our magnesium books.

Magnesium research continues to show the enormous benefits of this mineral, as you will see, and yet magnesium deficiency is still widespread. Large commercial farms have not seen fit to add magnesium-rich fertilizer to depleted soil, and people continue to eat magnesium-deficient foods made even more deficient by processing and cooking.

One bright light on the horizon was a 2006 World Health Organization (WHO) symposium, held in Baltimore, called "Calcium and Magnesium in Drinking Water." The WHO's acknowledgment of the importance of magnesium in health brings us closer to solving the magnesium deficiency problem we face. Paul Mason, of the Healthy Water Association, summarized the conference:

I.   There is consensus that most of the world's people are deficient in magnesium and calcium, resulting in vast numbers of deaths and debilitating illnesses worldwide.

II. There seemed to be agreement that there are only four ways of delivering adequate dietary magnesium to the global population:

A. Advising everyone on earth to take pills for magnesium and calcium. Nothing like this has ever been done, requiring behavior modification and decades of expensive advertising and promotion, which often fails. This route is very unlikely on a global level but practical on an individual level.

B. Advising everyone on earth to change their choices of foods to get more calcium and magnesium. This is another route that requires behavior modification and will likely fail on a global level but can be implemented on an individual level.

C. Adding calcium and magnesium to tap water. Most people feel this would be very wasteful since 99 percent of tap water is not used for drinking, and calcium especially can build up as scale in plumbing. Fortifying tap water is therefore very unlikely.

D. Requiring bottlers to add the optimal calcium and magnesium to bottled products might be our best option. WHO will study this problem and make a recommendation in 2008 and is likely to choose this alternative.

When I asked Mason if any countries were supplementing their water supply with magnesium, he said there is one practice that is noteworthy and which could be expanded. It has to do with desalinating seawater to make it fit for human use as drinking water. "As I understand it, all the countries that use reverse osmosis of seawater add back 1 percent seawater to prevent pipe corrosion caused by excessive softness. This amount of seawater will yield about 15 mg/L magnesium and 25 mg/L calcium. It varies around the world. I think Singapore and numerous Arab countries use reverse osmosis, and the list is steadily growing."

It may be decades before we see magnesium supplied in our drinking water; however, the WHO may encourage bottled water manufacturers to add this nutrient to their product. In the meantime, we can assess our own requirements and make sure we are doing all we can to keep our bodies supplied with the magnesium we need. To help in this regard, this expanded edition of *The Magnesium Miracle* offers specific recommendations on the best-absorbed forms of magnesium and a magnesium eating plan to help you obtain optimal levels of magnesium you need for your health.

INTRODUCTION

Do you know that most of us today are suffering from certain dangerous diet deficiencies which cannot be remedied until depleted soils from which our food comes are brought into proper mineral balance? The alarming fact is that foods (fruits, vegetables and grains) now being raised on millions of acres of land that no longer contain enough of certain minerals are starving us—no matter how much of them we eat. The truth is that our foods vary enormously in value, and some of them aren't worth eating as food. Our physical well-being is more directly dependent upon the minerals we take into our systems than upon calories or vitamins or upon the precise proportions of starch, protein or carbohydrates we consume. Laboratory tests prove that the fruits, the vegetables, the grains, the eggs, and even the milk and the meats of today are not what they were a few generations ago. No man today can eat enough fruits and vegetables to supply his stomach with the mineral salts he requires for perfect health, because his stomach isn't big enough to hold them! And we are turning into a nation of big stomachs.

—From the 74th Congress, 2nd session,
Senate document no. 264, 1936

It is hard to believe that this Senate document about mineral deficiency was written as long ago as 1936. Today farmlands are even more mineral-deficient and fertilizers still don't fully replace those minerals.

You only have to look at the *Journal of the American College of Nutrition*'s December 2004 issue to see our current dietary dilemma. A study by the U.S. Department of Agriculture on the nutritional status of forty-three garden crops assessed the level of protein, calcium, phosphorus, iron, riboflavin, and ascorbic acid. Researchers compared nutrient levels from 1950 with present values.

Remember, 1950 is fourteen years after the Senate document that claimed there were already significant deficiencies in our food supply. However, from 1950 to 2004, there was a further decline in nutrients in these crops, ranging from 6 percent for protein to 38 percent for riboflavin (a B vitamin).

The researchers admitted that this study raised significant questions about how modern agriculture practices are affecting food crops. One researcher said, "Perhaps more worrisome would be declines in nutrients we could not study because they were not reported in 1950—magnesium, zinc, vitamin B_6, vitamin E and dietary fiber, not to mention phytochemicals." The lead author of the paper, Dr. Donald Davis, hoped that "our paper will encourage additional studies in which old and new crop varieties are studied side-by-side and measured by modern methods."

My hope is different: that people will acknowledge the continuing decline of both our soil and the nutrient content of our foods and do something to repair those losses—not merely do further studies!

Magnesium is one of the most depleted minerals, yet one of the most important. We imagine that medicine has advanced to the stage of miracle cures, yet it's not technology that we're lacking but basic nutrients that power our bodies and give us our health.

Quick-fix medical solutions are all around us via television, the Internet, radio, and infomercials. In a world of rapid change, our bodies are going through peaks and crashes every day. We rely on double cappuccinos in the morning, a Power Bar for lunch, and an acupuncture treatment after work before we go to the gym for our energy hits. We're exhausting our natural physical stores of energy, straining our bodies' capacity to function and heal. Although we often can't change our workload, we can learn how to preserve and rebuild our energy levels naturally.

Magnesium regulates more than 325 enzymes in the body, the most important of which produce, transport, store, and utilize energy. Many aspects of cell metabolism are regulated by magnesium, such as DNA and RNA synthesis, cell growth, and cell reproduction. Magnesium also orchestrates the electric current that sparks through the miles of nerves in our body. Magnesium has numerous physiological roles, among which are control of nerve action, the activity of the heart, neuromuscular transmission, muscular contraction, vascular tone, blood pressure, and peripheral blood flow. Magnesium modulates and controls the entry and release of calcium from the cell, which determines muscular activity. Without magnesium, muscle and nerve functions are compromised and energy is diminished. We are operating with the power turned off. Muscular weakness, soft bones, anxiety, heart attacks, arrhythmia, and even seizures and convulsions can result.[1]

More than seventy-five years ago, scientists declared magnesium to be an essential mineral. Each year since then, research has revealed more ways in which magnesium is indispensable to life.[2] Yet it is continually being lost from the natural food supply. There has been a gradual decline of dietary magnesium in the United States, from a high of 500 mg/day at the turn of the century to barely 175–225 mg/day today.[3] The National Academy of Sciences has determined that most American men obtain about 80 percent of the recommended daily allowance (RDA) and women average only 70 percent.[4] In addition, most magnesium researchers find that the RDA is inadequate to prevent magnesium deficiency, making the above statistics of even more concern. In spite of this concern, few medical doctors are sounding the alarm, so it is left up to you to inform yourself and protect your health and that of your family.[5, 6, 7]

THE CLINICAL IMPACT OF MAGNESIUM DEFICIENCY

Magnesium was first discovered in huge deposits near a Greek city called Magnesia. Magnesium sulfate, known today as Epsom salts, was used in ancient times as a laxative, and still is to this day. A 1697 medical paper recommended magnesium, with some exaggerated unscientific enthusiasm, for conditions as varied as skin ulcers, depression, vertigo, heartburn, worms, kidney stones, jaundice, and gout. Most of these conditions are still treated with magnesium, and current research supports its use for a long list of ailments that you will read about in *The Magnesium Miracle.*

The amount of research on the topic of magnesium is staggering. To bring you the most current research and medical facts, I've sifted through thousands of pages of scientific studies, each of which begins with the acknowledgment that magnesium is of therapeutic value in treating a myriad of symptoms.

1. *Anxiety and panic attacks.* Magnesium normally helps keep adrenal stress hormones under control.

2. *Asthma.* Both histamine production and bronchial spasms increase with magnesium deficiency.

3. *Blood clots.* Magnesium has an important role to play in preventing blood clots and keeping the blood thin—without any side effects.

4. *Bowel disease.* Magnesium deficiency slows down the bowel, causing constipation, which could lead to toxicity and malabsorption of nutrients as well as colitis.

5. *Cystitis.* Bladder spasms are worsened by magnesium deficiency.

6. *Depression.* Serotonin, which elevates mood, is dependent on magnesium. A magnesium-deficient brain is also more susceptible to allergens, foreign substances that in rare instances can cause symptoms similar to mental illness.

7. *Detoxification.* Magnesium is crucial for the removal of toxic substances and heavy metals such as aluminum and lead from the body.

8. *Diabetes.* Magnesium enhances insulin secretion, facilitating sugar metabolism. Without magnesium, insulin is not able to transfer glucose into cells. Glucose and insulin build up in the blood, causing various types of tissue damage.

9. *Fatigue.* Magnesium-deficient patients commonly experience fatigue because dozens of enzyme systems are underfunctioning. An early symptom of magnesium deficiency is fatigue.

10. *Heart disease.* Magnesium deficiency is common in people with heart disease. Magnesium is administered in hospitals for acute myocardial infarction and cardiac arrhythmia. Like any other muscle, the heart requires magnesium. Magnesium is also used to treat angina, or chest pain.

11. *Hypertension.* With insufficient magnesium, blood vessels may go into spasm and cholesterol may rise, both of which lead to blood pressure problems.

12. *Hypoglycemia.* Magnesium keeps insulin under control; without magnesium, episodes of low blood sugar can result.

13. *Insomnia.* Sleep-regulating melatonin production is disturbed without sufficient magnesium.

14. *Kidney disease.* Magnesium deficiency contributes to atherosclerotic kidney failure. Magnesium deficiency creates abnormal lipid levels and worsening blood sugar control in kidney transplant patients.

15. *Migraine.* Serotonin balance is magnesium-dependent. Deficiency of serotonin can result in migraine headaches and depression.

16. *Musculoskeletal conditions.* Fibrositis, fibromyalgia, muscle spasms, eye twitches, cramps, and chronic neck and back pain may be caused by magnesium deficiency and can be relieved with magnesium supplements.

17. *Nerve problems.* Magnesium alleviates peripheral nerve disturbances throughout the body, such as headaches, muscle contractions, gastrointestinal spasms, and calf, foot, and toe cramps. It is also used in treating the central nervous system symptoms of vertigo and confusion.

18. *Obstetrical and gynecological problems.* Magnesium helps prevent premenstrual syndrome and dysmenorrhea (cramping pain during menses), is important in the treatment of infertility, and alleviates premature contractions, preeclampsia, and eclampsia in pregnancy. Intravenous magnesium is given in obstetrical wards for pregnancy-induced hypertension and to lessen the risk of cerebral palsy and sudden infant death

syndrome (SIDS). Magnesium should be a required supplement for pregnant women.

19. *Osteoporosis.* Use of calcium with vitamin D to enhance calcium absorption without a balancing amount of magnesium causes further magnesium deficiency, which triggers a cascade of events leading to bone loss.

20. *Raynaud's syndrome.* Magnesium helps relax the spastic blood vessels that cause pain and numbness of the fingers.

21. *Tooth decay.* Magnesium deficiency causes an unhealthy balance of phosphorus and calcium in saliva, which damages teeth.

Drugs such as painkillers, diuretics, antibiotics, and cortisone, many of which are inappropriately used for the aforementioned conditions, further deplete magnesium and other minerals, allowing symptoms to get completely out of control. Surgery, malnutrition, third-degree burns, serious injuries, pancreatic inflammation, liver disease, malabsorption disorders, diabetes, hormonal imbalance, and cancer are all seriously stressful medical conditions requiring increased amounts of magnesium.

MY HISTORY WITH MAGNESIUM

In my second year of medical school, I was observing in the obstetrics ward when a young woman in the last stage of labor developed rapidly elevating blood pressure and began convulsing. This was a true medical emergency. Already skeptical about the antihypertensive and anticonvulsant drugs, which had so many side effects and variable results, I wondered what could possibly work that would not be dangerous for the baby. But clearly, this woman needed something both powerful and effective. The attending physician called out for an ampule of magnesium sulfate and immediately injected it into the patient's IV. Within minutes the woman's convulsions had ceased and her blood pressure was returning to normal. I was amazed, and I've never forgotten that miracle of magnesium, which also reinforced my belief that there are safe, effective alternatives to prescription drugs for pain and chronic disease. In addition to my medical school training, I voraciously read all I could find on nutrition and alternative medicine. I even studied acupuncture. Immediately after medical school I embarked upon my naturopathic training. In thirteen years of treating patients and thirteen years as a researcher, writer, and consultant, I have frequently found myself acting as an educator, passing on the knowledge of simple, safe treatments and supplements that really work, including magnesium.

MY HOPE FOR THIS BOOK

Magnesium is not some wonder drug touted by a pharmaceutical company in an aggressive marketing campaign. It is a simple element, a mineral vital to life and health, and easily obtained. The more I have learned about magnesium, the more convinced I am that doctors are missing a huge opportunity by not making it one of their drugs of choice. I hope that this rich story of magnesium will assist in improving your health and at the same time provide a valuable resource that you can share with your doctor.

THE
MAGNESIUM
MIRACLE

PART ONE

THE HISTORY OF MAGNESIUM

===

CHAPTER ONE

THE CASE FOR MAGNESIUM

Mary joked that she felt as though she were constantly being run over by a slow-moving bus. Cramping in her legs startled her awake at night, making her an insomniac, and she had heart palpitations daily. Her doctor also found that she had high blood sugar. It wasn't bad enough for her to need injections of insulin, but he prescribed pills to try to stimulate more insulin production. Finally, frightening panic attacks came out of nowhere and made this vibrant, fun-loving woman afraid to go outside.

To try to relieve her leg cramps, Mary began taking calcium at night, having read that it was good for cramps and sleep. At first, the calcium seemed to help, but after a week or two, the pains got worse. If she yawned and stretched in bed, her calf muscles would seize up and catapult her to the floor, where she would lie frantically massaging her muscles to try to release the spasm. All the next day, she would limp about with a very tender, bruised feeling in her calf.

Although Mary's heart palpitations had improved somewhat after she'd given up her three cups of coffee a day, they too resumed after a few weeks. Every time the palpitations occurred, which was several times a day, they made her cough slightly and catch her breath. She found it frightening, even though her doctor said her stress tests for heart disease were fine and she didn't need further testing with an angiogram.

Both Mary's parents had had adult-onset diabetes, and Mary knew that she should watch her diet, but she was overweight and craved sugary and high-carbohydrate foods that were hard to resist. When the panic attacks hit on top of everything else, Mary knew she had to seek help, and came to my office. She was only fifty-three, far too young to be feeling so bad, and was worried about her future health.

Sam was only forty-nine and experiencing chest pains. At first, he thought they were indigestion, but sometimes the pains would occur in the middle of the night. Concerned, he went to a cardiologist, who found two slightly blocked arteries, not serious enough for bypass surgery. Sam's cholesterol was somewhat elevated, as was his blood pressure, which he attributed to his high-stress occupation and the fact that he had not exercised regularly for the past six months, when he was sidelined with back pain. The cardiologist observed that his arterial blockage would almost inevitably worsen over time and eventually necessitate surgery. The doctor offered him medication for his high cholesterol, told him not to eat butter or eggs, and gave him nitroglycerine to take whenever he had the pain. If the symptoms got worse, he would prescribe other medications. Sam couldn't imagine having to wait to get worse before doing something about his chest pain; he knew there must be something more he could do to avoid surgery, and came to me for advice.

At thirty-five, Jan had actually begun to look forward to going through menopause. That's how bad her PMS symptoms were. As soon as those horrible feelings lifted, she was hit by the sledgehammer of menstrual cramps. She also had migraines, which for years had come before her period but now were occurring once or twice a week. She was so miserable that she was considering a complete hysterectomy, with removal of her hormone-producing ovaries, but wondered whether the migraines, since they were happening all month, were not actually hormonal.

Different as their symptoms are, Mary, Sam, and Jan all suffer from magnesium deficiency. While women and men seem equally susceptible to magnesium deficiency, women, pound for pound, have less magnesium. They have fewer circulating red blood cells, which carry magnesium, and so perhaps less magnesium available, but they seem to utilize the magnesium they do have more efficiently than men.

There are a few other gender differences. Because of magnesium's effect on hormonal regulation and vice versa, women appear to have more problems with low magnesium because they can suffer deficiencies during pregnancy, when breast-feeding, with premenstrual syndrome (PMS), and with dysmenorrhea (painful periods). Osteoporosis, which affects more women than men, is evidence of a deficiency of both calcium and magnesium. An overactive thyroid, which afflicts more women than men, increases the metabolic rate, which uses up magnesium-requiring ATP (adenosine triphosphate—the energy packets made in each cell in the body). Without magnesium, ATP would not be produced. However, women's efficient use of magnesium may explain why prior to menopause they are protected from heart attacks.

Let's follow Mary, Sam, and Jan and see how they overcame their magnesium deficiencies.

When Mary visited me, I charted her health history in detail, according to procedures commonly used by naturopathic doctors, and found several symptoms of magnesium deficiency. In her case it had been made even worse by too much calcium, however, so simple magnesium supplementation wouldn't be enough for Mary. Her diet and lifestyle needed a complete overhaul. I explained that calcium appears to help leg cramps, at least initially, because excess calcium forces magnesium to be released from storage sites. But if someone is magnesium-deficient, the excess calcium can begin to cause more problems.

I gave Mary a list of magnesium-rich foods that she needed to start eating, which included nuts, beans, greens, and seeds such as sunflower and pumpkin. Mary realized that she'd been avoiding almost all of these foods: she thought nuts were fattening, beans gave her gas, and greens never seemed fresh enough at the supermarket. She had never even thought about eating seeds.

After a week of enthusiastically eating a lot more magnesium-rich foods, Mary felt somewhat better. To make sure she could get fresh organic greens regularly, she tracked down a local community-supported agriculture (CSA) program and bought a share in a neighboring organic farm. Mary also learned how to soak and cook beans to prevent them from causing gas, and began eating nuts and seeds rich in magnesium and healthy oils, such as almonds, walnuts, pecans, sunflower seeds, and pumpkin seeds.

After her second visit I recommended that Mary begin taking magnesium supplements. Starting with a dosage of 200 mg a day, we added another 200 mg every two days to build slowly to 600 mg. I cautioned her that it could take months to eliminate magnesium deficiency symptoms and that not all her symptoms would necessarily respond. Mary, excited by the improvement she felt by just increasing magnesium-rich foods, expressed impatience and wanted to know if she should have intravenous magnesium to saturate her tissues more quickly. I explained that IV magnesium would indeed do just that, but perhaps a simpler and less expensive way would be to spray magnesium oil on her body and use it regularly in baths, including foot baths. Within one month, Mary was singing the praises of magnesium. Her palpitations and panic attacks had disappeared. Her cravings for sweets were fewer, she was able to control her blood sugar with diet alone, and tests for blood sugar were normal. Her leg cramps were gone, and with them her insomnia. At three months we added calcium along with magnesium so that she would not develop an imbalance of the two. Mary's internist was quite surprised at her improved health and told her to keep up the good work with her diet and supplements.

Sam had an inquiring mind, and I encouraged him to start reading about heart disease and magnesium. He found that up to 30 percent of angina (chest pain) patients do not have badly blocked arteries but may be suffering from an electrical imbalance that is driven by mineral deficiency, most commonly magnesium.[1] An astonishing 40 to 60 percent of sudden deaths from heart attack may occur in the complete absence of any prior artery blockage, clot formation, or heart rhythm abnormalities, most likely from spasms in the arteries (magnesium is a natural antispasmodic).[2, 3, 4, 5] Moreover, he found that magnesium deficiency has been linked to sudden cardiac death. Sam didn't want to wait around for that to happen to him; he was determined to find out what was causing his problem and treat the cause. The more he read, the more intrigued he became. When he read that magnesium deficiency is also associated with muscle pain, especially back pain, that really got his attention, since he had begun having back pain four or five months before he developed chest pain.[6]

With a packet of information on magnesium, Sam went back to his cardiologist. After waiting impatiently for the doctor a full thirty minutes, a nurse took Sam's blood pressure; it was elevated, even though at home it was usually only a few points above normal. (Doctor-induced hypertension is commonly reported by patients.) After hearing the blood pressure reading from his nurse, the cardiologist swept into Sam's room and immediately began talking about blood pressure medication. Sam countered with magnesium. The cardiologist visibly cooled and said that magnesium was used to control hypertension that occurred in pregnant women because there were no side effects, but that there were plenty of effective drugs for everyone else. When Sam said he would rather not have side effects either, the cardiologist gathered up his file and told him to come back when he was ready to take medications for his heart disease.

When Sam came back to see me, he was still pretty upset by this encounter; he didn't like the specialist refusing to discuss a possible magnesium deficiency as part of the picture. Sam and I agreed that magnesium seemed the best treatment for him to initiate at this time since he was not willing to take medications.

Sam began adding magnesium to his diet by eating magnesium-rich foods. After a week he felt much calmer, but he still had chest and back pain. So he added magnesium supplements, and in about three months he felt almost normal.

Among the studies Sam read was one that looked at the correspondence between type A personalities and magnesium deficiency. From the description, Sam realized he was a type A, an aggressive guy who lived on adrenaline, time pressure, and stress. This type of behavior drains the body of magnesium and can lead to disorders such as heart disease, muscle spasms, hypersensitivity, and irritability.[7] Prolonged psychological stress raises adrenaline, the stress hormone, which depletes magnesium.[8] Both Sam's back and chest pain would hit when he was under stress. So Sam worked on ways to control his stress and added more magnesium when he knew he couldn't avoid it. On days when he exercised, Sam added an extra 200 mg of magnesium to his regime, since sweat loss during heavy exercise (cycling and jogging) and working in the heat deplete magnesium. Just drinking water won't replace all the minerals lost. By paying attention to the many factors that affected his mind-body health, Sam lowered his cholesterol and stress levels and reduced his chance of a heart attack and of needing surgery to unblock his arteries.

Jan heard that yoga might help her PMS and painful periods, and she really needed to learn to relax, so she took classes at a local health club. The teacher also ran regular detox and cooking classes, which Jan decided to join when she realized she didn't have to "give up everything" and become a vegetarian. One of the first things Jan learned in the detox class was the importance of having regular bowel movements. Jan was lucky if she had one a week. If the bowel doesn't empty once a day, toxins can be reabsorbed back into the body from the colon. The longer debris sits in the colon, the more fluid is reabsorbed, making stools more solid and difficult to pass. PMS and endometriosis, which causes painful periods, are considered by some natural-health experts to worsen with constipation and toxicity.[9]

During cooking classes, Jan faced the fact that she was a junk food addict. Magnesium is necessary in hundreds of enzymes in the body but is almost totally lost during the processing of packaged and fast foods. The older women in her class were suffering from a variety of problems that included cancer, heart disease, and osteoporosis. Is that how she would end up in ten or twenty years if she didn't take care of her health now? Learning how many basic nutrients she lacked in her diet made her marvel that she wasn't even more ill. Her new diet included greens, beans, nuts, and seeds, which cleared up her constipation and almost eliminated her PMS and painful periods. When she came to see me on the advice of her yoga teacher, it was clear she was on the right track. I recommended that she begin taking a magnesium supplement along with calcium and a multiple vitamin; with all her lifestyle changes, she felt like a new person.

MAGNESIUM, THE SPARK OF LIFE

In a poetic reference to magnesium's crucial role in evolution, Dr. Jerry Aikawa of the University of Colorado calls magnesium the ur-mineral, the most important mineral to man and all other living organisms.[10] It is critical to the metabolic processes of lowly one-celled living organisms and is the second most abundant element inside human cells. Magnesium existed at the beginning of life and was involved with all aspects of cell production and growth. When plants evolved to use the sun as their energy source, magnesium played a pivotal role in the development of chlorophyll. So in both plants and animals, magnesium became an essential mineral involved in hundreds of enzyme processes affecting every aspect of life.

Presently, seventeen minerals are considered essential for human life, and it is quite possible that more minerals will be found to be indispensable as we take more time to study life's mineral connection. Ninety-nine percent of the body's mineral content is made up of seven macrominerals: sodium, potassium, calcium, phosphorus, chlorine, sulfur, and magnesium. The other 1 percent comprises ten trace minerals. As with most minerals, the element magnesium occurs in nature combined with other elements. It joins naturally with sulfur to make Epsom salts (magnesium sulfate), with carbon to make magnesium carbonate, and with calcium to make dolomite. Magnesium is also found in partnership with silica in talc and asbestos. Like calcium, it is an alkaline mineral, which neutralizes acid, and some magnesium compounds are antacids used to treat heartburn.

My first encounter with magnesium was in high school chemistry. Each student was given a thin strip of magnesium and told to light one end carefully. The previous week we had learned that magnesium is the eighth most abundant element, constituting approximately 2 percent of the earth's crust and 1.14 percent of seawater. By comparison, calcium makes up 3 percent of the earth's crust but only 0.05 percent of seawater. There are 4–6 tsp (20–28 g or 2 oz) of magnesium in the body, comprising about 0.05 percent of the body's weight. This information in no way prepared us for the dynamic effect of lighting the magnesium strip. It flared up like an electric sparkler and disappeared in a flash. This incendiary property serves as an important reminder of magnesium's versatility as the spark of life, constantly igniting metabolic reactions throughout the body.

THE BODY IS ELECTRIC

The impulses for any and all movement in the body arise from electrical transmission. These microcurrents of electricity that pass along the nerves were first measured in 1966. Scientists soon discovered that the conductor for these bodily electrical currents was calcium and that magnesium was necessary to maintain the proper level of calcium in the blood.[11] More recent research indicates that calcium enters the cells by way of calcium channels that are jealously guarded by magnesium. Magnesium, at a concentration 10,000 times greater than that of calcium in the cells, allows only a certain amount of calcium to enter to create the necessary electrical transmission, and then immediately helps to eject the calcium once the work is done. Why? If calcium accumulates in the cell, it causes hyperexcitibility and calcification and disrupts cell function. Too much calcium entering cells can cause symptoms of heart disease (such as angina, high blood pressure, and arrhythmia), asthma, or headaches. Magnesium is nature's calcium channel blocker.[12, 13, 14]

About 60–65 percent of all our magnesium is housed in

our bones and teeth. The remaining 35–40 percent is found in the rest of the body, including muscle and tissue cells and body fluids. The highest concentrations are in the heart and brain cells, so it is no wonder that the major symptoms of magnesium deficiency affect the heart and brain. These are also the two organs that have considerable electrical activity, measured by EKG (electrocardiogram) and EEG (electroencephalogram). Our blood contains only *1 percent* of the body's total magnesium.

Magnesium mostly works inside our tissue cells, bonding with ATP to produce energy packets for our body's vital force. Not enough can be said about the importance of this energy-producing function of magnesium. The combination of ATP and magnesium triggers production of all the body's protein structures by revving up messenger RNA. This combination is also a requirement for the production of DNA, our genetic code. Both basic building blocks of life, RNA and DNA, are dependent on ATP/magnesium to maintain stable genes.[15] In addition to its stabilizing effect on DNA and the structure of chromosomes, ATP/magnesium is an essential cofactor in almost all enzyme systems involved in the processing of DNA. Research shows that without sufficient magnesium, DNA synthesis becomes sluggish.

WHAT DOES MAGNESIUM DO?

Magnesium's hundreds of activities in the human body can be divided into five essential categories:[16]

1. Magnesium is a cofactor assisting enzymes in catalyzing most chemical reactions in the body, including temperature regulation.
2. Magnesium produces and transports energy.

3. Magnesium is necessary for the synthesis of protein.
4. Magnesium helps to transmit nerve signals.
5. Magnesium helps to relax muscles.

1. COFACTOR IN CHEMICAL REACTIONS

Enzymes are protein molecules that stimulate every chemical reaction in the body. Magnesium is required to make hundreds of these enzymes work and assists with thousands of others.

2. PRODUCING AND TRANSPORTING ENERGY

Magnesium and the B-complex vitamins are excellent examples of energy nutrients, because they activate enzymes that control digestion, absorption, and the utilization of proteins, fats, and carbohydrates. Because magnesium is involved with hundreds of enzymatic reactions throughout the body, deficiency can affect every aspect of life and cause a score of symptoms. Of the 325 magnesium-dependent enzymes, the most important enzyme reaction involves the creation of energy by activating adenosine triphosphate (ATP), the fundamental energy storage molecule of the body. ATP may be what the Chinese refer to as *qi* or life force. Magnesium is required for the body to produce and store energy. Without magnesium there is no energy, no movement, no life. It is that simple.

3. SYNTHESIZING PROTEIN

Magnesium is used in synergy with dozens of other vitamins and minerals to create structural components of the body. Under the direction of magnesium, enzymes and nutrients modify the building blocks from food to create the body. Without magnesium, there is no body. RNA and DNA, which contain the genetic blueprints for the formation of all the protein molecules in the body, are also dependent on magnesium.

4. TRANSMITTING NERVE SIGNALS

Magnesium permits a small amount of calcium to enter a nerve cell, just enough to allow electrical transmission along the nerves to and from the brain, then forces it back outside. Even our thoughts, via brain neurons, are dependent on magnesium.

5. RELAXING MUSCLES

Calcium causes contraction in skeletal muscle fibers, and magnesium causes relaxation. When there is too much calcium and insufficient magnesium inside a cell, you can get sustained muscle contraction: twitches, spasms, and even convulsions. Smooth muscles directed by too much calcium and insufficient magnesium can tighten the bronchial tract, causing asthma; cause cramping in the uterus and painful periods; and cause spasms in blood vessels, resulting in hypertension.

WHO IS DEFICIENT?

The most frequent questions I'm asked about magnesium is "How do I know I need more magnesium?" and "Should I take magnesium supplements?" I have come to the conclusion that everyone could benefit from extra supplementation. However, there is a long list of possible symptoms and behaviors that can identify your need for magnesium. The following 100 factors in 68 categories can help you recognize magnesium deficiency. There's no way of knowing how many factors correlate with any one person's magnesium deficiency, but if you find yourself ticking off a few dozen, you may want see how many of your symptoms improve when you take magnesium supplements.

1. Alcohol intake—more than seven drinks per week
2. Anger
3. Angina
4. Anxiety
5. Apathy
6. Arrhythmia of the heart
7. Asthma
8. Blood tests
   a. Low calcium
   b. Low potassium
   c. Low magnesium
9. Bowel problems
   a. Undigested fat in stool
   b. Constipation
   c. Diarrhea
   d. Alternating constipation and diarrhea
   e. IBS
   f. Crohn's
   g. Colitis
10. Brain trauma
11. Bronchitis, chronic
12. Caffeine (coffee, tea, chocolate), more than three servings per day
13. Chronic fatigue syndrome
14. Cold extremities
15. Concentration difficulties
16. Confusion
17. Convulsions
18. Depression
19. Diabetes
    a. Type I
    b. Type II
    c. Gestational diabetes
20. Fibromyalgia

21. Food intake imbalances
    a. Limited in green leafy vegetables, seeds, and fresh fruit
    b. High protein
22. Food cravings
    a. Carbohydrates
    b. Chocolate
    c. Salt
    d. Junk food
23. Gagging or choking on food
24. Headaches
25. Heart disease
26. Heart—rapid rate
27. High blood pressure
28. Homocysteinuria
29. Hyperactivity
30. Hyperventilation
31. Infertility
32. Insomnia
33. Irritability
34. Kidney stones
35. Medications
    a. Digitalis
    b. Diuretics
    c. Antibiotics
    d. Steroids
    e. Oral contraceptives
    f. Indomethacin
    g. Cisplatin
    h. Amphotericin B
    i. Cholestyramine
    j. Synthetic estrogens
36. Memory impairment
37. Mercury amalgam dental fillings

38. Menstrual pain and cramps
39. Migraines
40. Mineral supplements
    a. Take calcium without magnesium
    b. Take zinc without magnesium
    c. Take iron without magnesium
41. Mitral valve prolapse
42. Muscle cramps or spasms
43. Muscle twitching or tics
44. Muscle weakness
45. Numbness of hands or feet
46. Osteoporosis
47. Paranoia
48. Parathyroid hyperactivity
49. PMS
50. Polycystic ovarian disease
51. Pregnancy
    a. Currently pregnant
    b. Pregnant within one year
    c. History of preeclampsia or eclampsia
    d. Postpartum depression
    e. Have a child with cerebral palsy
52. Radiation therapy, recent
53. Raynaud's syndrome
54. Restlessness
55. Sexual energy diminished
56. Shortness of breath
57. Smoking
58. Startled easily by noise
59. Stressful life or circumstances
60. Stroke
61. Sugar, high intake daily
62. Syndrome X
63. Thyroid hyperactivity

64. Tingling of hands or feet
65. Transplants
    a. Kidney
    b. Liver
66. Tremor of the hands
67. Water that contains the following
    a. Fluoride
    b. Chlorine
    c. Calcium
68. Wheezing

THE DANCE OF CALCIUM AND MAGNESIUM

Calcium and magnesium share equal importance in our bodies. Appropriating Newton's law of physics that says for every action there is an equal and opposite reaction, neither calcium or magnesium can act without eliciting a reaction from the other. At the biochemical level, magnesium and calcium are known to act antagonistically toward each other. Many enzymes whose activities critically depend on a sufficient amount of intracellular magnesium (10,000 times more than calcium) will be detrimentally affected by small increases in levels of cellular calcium. Growth of cells, cell division, and intermediary metabolism are also absolutely dependent on the availability of magnesium, which can be compromised if excess calcium is present.[17]

To understand how you can create a calcium/magnesium imbalance in your own body, try this experiment in your kitchen. Crush a calcium pill and see how much dissolves in 1 oz of water. Then crush a magnesium pill and slowly stir it into the calcium water. When you introduce the magnesium, the remaining calcium dissolves; it becomes more water-soluble. The same thing happens in your bloodstream, heart, brain, kidneys, and all the other tissues in your body. If you don't have enough magnesium to help keep calcium dissolved, you may end up with calcium-excess muscle spasms, fibromyalgia, hardening of the arteries, calcium deposits, and even dental cavities. Another scenario plays out in the kidneys and bladder. If there is too much calcium in the kidneys and not enough magnesium to dissolve it, you can get kidney stones. Calcium deposited throughout the bladder can make it rigid, lower its capacity, and lead to frequent urination.

All muscles, including the heart and blood vessels, contain more magnesium than calcium. If magnesium is deficient, calcium floods the smooth muscle cells of the blood vessels and causes spasms leading to constricted blood vessels and therefore higher blood pressure, arterial spasm, angina, and heart attack.[18] A proper balance of magnesium in relation to calcium can prevent these symptoms. Calcium excess, stimulating the cells in the muscular layer of the temporal arteries (located over the temples) can cause migraine headaches. Excess calcium can constrict the smooth muscle surrounding the small airways of the lung, causing restricted breathing and asthma. Finally, too much calcium, without the protective effect of magnesium, can irritate delicate nerve cells of the brain. Cells that are irritated by calcium fire electrical impulses repeatedly, depleting their energy stores and causing cell death.

THE CALCIUM DISTRACTION

The irony of the calcium-magnesium story is that without magnesium calcium will not work properly. Both our current diet and tendency to oversupplement with calcium, however, make getting enough magnesium almost impossible. Research shows that the ratio of calcium to magnesium in the Paleolithic or caveman diet—the ancient diet that evolved with our bodies—was 1:1, compared with a 5:1 to 15:1 ratio in present-day diets.[19] With an average of ten times more calcium than magnesium in our current diet, there is no doubt about widespread magnesium deficiency in modern times.

The emphasis on calcium supplementation has diverted our attention from any other mineral, even though all minerals are crucial to the proper functioning of the body. In our society we tend to look for "the best," "the most important," "the star," and forget that it takes a team and teamwork to get anything accomplished, including body processes. Calcium, because it is the most abundant mineral in the body, therefore became "the star." Even though research has accumulated on magnesium over the past four decades, it has never been adequately publicized and discussed.

≡

CHAPTER TWO

MAGNESIUM: THE MISSING MINERAL

A 1988 U.S. government study concluded that the standard American diet failed to provide the daily requirement of magnesium.[1] That was almost two decades ago, and you can be sure that most people get even less today, when junk food makes up 27 percent of our diet. Mildred Seelig, M.D., and many other magnesium experts have also come to the inescapable conclusion that the typical American diet, which is rich in fat, sugar, salt, synthetic vitamin D, phosphates, protein, and supplemented calcium, not only is deficient in magnesium but actually *increases* the need for magnesium in the body.

Unfortunately, it is impossible to find studies that tell us the actual incidence of magnesium deficiency. This stems from there being no accepted medical standard for measuring whole-body magnesium status. As will be discussed in Chapter 16, blood testing for magnesium relies on inadequate measurements since only 1 percent of the body's magnesium is in the blood and only 40 percent in the tissues. The National Academy of Sciences found that *most* Americans are possibly magnesium-deficient. When men obtain only 80 percent of the minimum requirement of magnesium to run innumerable body functions and women at 70 percent get even less of what they absolutely need, then our bodies are just not able to function properly.[2]

Let's look at some of the reasons you may be lacking in magnesium—and it begins with what's missing from the soil.

MAGNESIUM-DEFICIENT SOIL

The mineral depletion of our farmland quoted from the 1936 Senate document in the introduction to *The Magnesium Miracle* is probably the most important reason why most Americans are magnesium-deficient. Unfortunately, the issue of depleted soils has not been addressed in America. As Kirkpatrick Sale expressed in *The Nation*, after World War II it only got worse.

> When U.S. industrialism turned to agriculture after World War II, for example, it went at it with all that it had just learned on the battlefield, using tractors modeled on wartime tanks to cut up vast fields, crop-dusters modeled on wartime planes to spray poisons, and pesticides and herbicides developed from wartime chemical weapons and defoliants to destroy unwanted species. It was a war on the land, sweeping and sophisticated as modern mechanization can be, capable of depleting topsoil at the rate of 3 billion tons a year and water at the rate of 10 billion gallons a year. It could be no other way: If a nation like this beats its swords into plowshares, they will still be violent and deadly tools.
>
> —*The Nation*, June 5, 1995

DEAD SOIL

Kirkpatrick Sale talks about the war waged on the land and all species on it by farmers lured into believing that killing weeds and pests was far superior to living in harmony with nature.

The whole experiment backfired when it became clear that the poisons could not be controlled—they killed indiscriminately. Without living worms and nitrogen-fixing rhizobacteria, the soil became dead. Worms break up the earth, leaving their own form of compost behind, and without this activity the soil becomes hard and nonporous. Bacteria in the soil make it possible for plants to absorb certain nutrients, and without their action plants are weaker and less nutritious.

Observing animals can teach us important lessons about our environment—if we only listen. One man who did was André Voisin, a French biochemist and farmer born in 1903. In 1963 Voisin wrote a book called *Grass Tetany*. Grass tetany is a metabolic disease of cattle and goats caused by a deficiency of magnesium in the soil. When animals eat magnesium-deficient grass they develop irritability, staggering, tremors, and spasms. Most dramatically, the animals fall down in convulsions at sudden loud noises or if they are frightened or excited. Voisin reported that in the 1930s magnesium deficiency had been proven to be the cause of grass tetany, since low levels of magnesium were found in suffering animals and the condition was miraculously reversed by injections of magnesium.

Chapter 1 of Voisin's book says it all: "Modern Farming Methods Favour the Development of Grass Tetany." In his career as a farmer, Voisin observed that "intensive grazing" and the overuse of mineral-deficient commercial fertilizers were common practices. At the time, Voisin identified Holland as the country that used the most commercial fertilizer on its pastures and also suffered the most grass tetany.

A potassium product called potash has been the fertilizer of choice since the 1930s. It's cheap, easily obtained, and readily absorbed by plants. In fact, it is so easily taken up by plants that when there is an abundance of potassium they favor its absorption above magnesium and calcium, which are relatively harder to absorb. Crops grown with excessive amounts of potash have a low content of magnesium and calcium and high potassium levels. However, you would never know that since there is no minimum amount of minerals required in our grains, fruits, or vegetables—the nutrients in such foods are not routinely measured and never labeled.

Even if the magnesium content of soil is high, using potassium fertilizer can prevent its absorption into the plant. But because most agricultural land in America has been overworked for decades and fertilizers don't replace this important mineral, magnesium is rarely found in our soils.

SOIL EROSION

Paul Mason, owner of a magnesium-rich spring in California, reminds us that magnesium is also susceptible to being leached from cultivated soil.[3] Based on a measure of the dissolved magnesium in the Mississippi River, estimates are that the annual loss of magnesium from midwestern soils is an incredible 7.1 million kg at least, and likely more if the magnesium in undissolved dirt carried by the river is included.

BURNING OFF MAGNESIUM WITH ACID RAIN

Acid rain provides yet another attack on the magnesium in soil; it occurs in industrial and urban areas that experience excessive air pollution. Atmospheric scientist William Grant, during his study of air pollution, concluded that an accumulation of acid rain, which contains nitric acid, can change the chemistry of the soil in which trees grow.[4] This abnormal soil acidity creates a reaction with calcium and magnesium in the soil to neutralize the excess nitric acid. He found that eventually these minerals are depleted, leaving the nitric acid to react with the aluminum oxide in the soil. The reactive aluminum builds up, replaces the calcium and magnesium in the plant, and makes it difficult for the plant to survive.

Calcium is beneficial to trees and plants because it strengthens the walls of the cells that combine to shape the tree, so without it plants weaken. Magnesium is an essential component of the chlorophyll necessary for photosynthesis, during which organic chemicals are produced during exposure to sunlight. While calcium and magnesium deficiency weakens the plant, the acid rain also provides more nitrates to the plants, causing them to grow faster. The lack of calcium and magnesium, however, means that this early growth cannot be supported, and the plants may be too weak to survive.

If we eat plants that are grown on soil contaminated with acid rain, they may be very deficient in calcium and magnesium. On the farm, soil acidity is tested, and if the soil is too acid it is usually treated with lime—a calcium oxide product. Treating with lime is another practice that can result in magnesium-deficient plants. You can read more about calcium-magnesium interactions on page 251.

DEFICIENT PRODUCE FROM DEFICIENT SOIL

When you walk into a grocery story and pick up your produce, for the most part you just want it to look nice. You reject bruised, wilted, or misshapen vegetables or fruit. This emphasis on superficial appearance, not nutritional content, is what drives the industry. There is no labeling law that requires that the level of magnesium be displayed prominently.

Foods that commonly contain magnesium are leafy green vegetables, nuts, seeds, and whole grains. However, unlike vitamins, which can be manufactured by plants if they have sufficient sunlight and water, minerals must be present in the soil to show up in plants. If there is no magnesium in the soil, plants will have none; they cannot manufacture it out of thin air. So don't believe it when someone says that you can get all your nutrients in a good, balanced diet. That may be true only if you eat organic food, and then only if the organic farmers use a full spectrum of nutrients in their fertilizer. I'm convinced that to get enough magnesium today, you need to take supplements.

PROCESSED FOOD LACKS MAGNESIUM

During the refining and processing of food, significant amounts of magnesium can be lost. The process of extracting oils from magnesium-rich nuts and seeds strips away this essential mineral. Nearly all the magnesium in grains is lost during the milling process when the bran and germ are removed from whole grain to make white flour. For example, one slice of whole-wheat bread holds on to 24 mg of the mineral, while a slice of white bread has only 6 mg. And yet magnesium is never considered in the fortification of refined foods. Finally, in the kitchen, when vegetables are boiled, magnesium leaches out into the water. Of note is the fact that less calcium than magnesium is lost due to food processing and cooking, making the average diet higher in calcium than magnesium.

PERCENTAGE OF MAGNESIUM LOST DURING FOOD PROCESSING

Refining of flour from wheat	80 percent
Polishing of rice	83 percent
Production of starch from corn	97 percent
Extraction of white sugar from molasses	99 percent

What can we do to defend our magnesium sources? It is best to buy organic foods, eat as many raw vegetables as possible, and when you do cook vegetables, quickly steam them for only a few minutes, until they are slightly cooked but still crisp. You must also save the nutrient-filled water to use as soup stock. Chapter 17 presents the Magnesium Eating Plan, through which you can add whole grains, nuts, seeds, and greens to your diet.

FLUORIDATED WATER BANISHES MAGNESIUM

Fluoridation of tap water is a disaster that threatens to afflict the population with an epidemic of arthritis and, by recent reports, cancer as well. While most of Europe and half of the United States have completely abandoned the use of fluoride in the water supply, it still remains in the other half of the United States, in toothpaste, and as a molecule in SSRI antidepressants such as Prozac. Fluoride seeks out minerals such as magnesium and binds with it, making magnesium unavailable to the body and unable to do its work. The magnesium fluoride mineral produced is called sellaite; it is almost insoluble and ends up taking the place of magnesium in hard tissues like bone and cartilage, but its brittleness makes the bone susceptible to fracture. The reduction in available magnesium causes a decrease in enzymatic action in the body.[5]

In addition to its interactions with magnesium, fluoride has other harmful effects in the body. When I interviewed Dr. Paul Connett from the Fluoride Action Network on a radio program in September 2005, he reported that Harvard grad student Elise Bassin, in her Ph.D. thesis, found a strong correlation between water fluoridation and osteosarcoma, a type of bone cancer. There was a 700 percent increase in osteosarcoma in young men if they were exposed to fluoridated water during their sixth to eighth years. And according to the U.S. Department of Health and Human Services, "subsets of the population may be unusually susceptible to the toxic effects of fluoride and its compounds. These populations include the elderly, people with magnesium deficiency, and people with cardiovascular and kidney problems."[6]

STOMACH ACID IS ESSENTIAL FOR MAGNESIUM ABSORPTION

Inefficient stomach digestion and intestinal absorption can lead to deficiencies of magnesium. What's worse, when magnesium is deficient, magnesium absorption is hindered even more.

When you are under serious physical or even emotional stress, your body might not produce sufficient stomach acid, which is required for digestion and for chemically changing minerals into an absorbable form. Minerals are usually bound to another substance to make a mineral complex; for example, magnesium bound to citric acid creates magnesium citrate, and bound to the amino acid taurine it makes magnesium taurate. When a magnesium complex hits the stomach, it needs an acidic environment to help break the two substances apart, leaving magnesium in the ionic form and ready for action in the body.

The elderly as well as people with arthritis, asthma, depression, diabetes, gallbladder disease, osteoporosis, or gum disease are often deficient in hydrochloric acid.[7] All these conditions are also associated with magnesium deficiency.

Another disruption to digestion is America's addiction to antacids—the number one over-the-counter drug family. Heartburn and indigestion, the result of bad eating habits, plague the nation. But the "cure" in this case is no better than the disease. The roiling and burning in the gut from sugary junk food and greasy fast food is being inappropriately blamed on *too much* stomach acid. In many cases, heartburn is due to sugar fermentation in the stomach and a backflow of pancreatic enzymes from the small intestine.[8] By neutralizing normal stomach acids, antacids make it impossible for us to absorb minerals or digest our food properly. Our magnesium can be even further depleted if we use calcium carbonate antacids because the calcium they contain causes more magnesium to be excreted.

It's also important to understand the grave effects low stomach acid and low magnesium have on calcium absorption. I've already talked about calcium's inability to dissolve in water, making it entirely dependent on stomach acid to put it into solution. However, when it leaves the stomach's highly acidic environment it enters the alkaline environment of the small intestine and precipitates out of solution unless sufficient magnesium is present. Without magnesium to keep it in solution, calcium quickly deposits in soft tissues throughout the body.

In the large intestine, it interferes with peristalsis (the waves of muscle contractions that push food through the bowels), which results in constipation. When calcium precipitates out in the kidneys and combines with phosphorous or oxalic acid, kidney stones are formed. Calcium can deposit in the lining of the bladder and prevent it from fully relaxing, and therefore from filling completely with urine. This leads to frequent urination problems, especially in older people.

Calcium can precipitate out of the blood and deposit in the lining of arteries, causing hardening of the arteries (arteriosclerosis). It can coat and stiffen cholesterol deposits (plaque) in the arteries, leading to atherosclerosis. This, in turn, can cause blood pressure to rise as well as increase the risk of heart attack and stroke. Calcium can even deposit in the brain. Many researchers are investigating it as a possible cause of dementia, Alzheimer's, and Parkinson's disease.

Calcium can deposit in the lining of the bronchial tubes and cause asthma symptoms. Calcium in the extracellular fluid can surround cells in body tissue (organs, muscles) and decrease the permeability of the cell membranes. This makes it increasingly more difficult for glucose (a very large molecule) to pass through the cell membrane to be converted into ATP (adenosine triphosphate) in the cells' mitochondria. High glucose levels created by excess calcium may be misdiagnosed as diabetes.

ABSORPTION OF DIETARY MAGNESIUM IS HINDERED

Magnesium is ultimately absorbed into the bloodstream from the small intestine. At the best of times, only about one-half (down to as little as one-third) of the magnesium that is contained in food and water is absorbed; the rest is eliminated in the stool or urine. A study reported in *Metabolism* used radioactive magnesium to trace the activities of the mineral in the body.[9] It was observed that, on a diet with an average amount of magnesium, 44 percent of the ingested radioactive magnesium was absorbed; on a low-magnesium diet, 76 percent was absorbed; and on a high-magnesium diet, only 24 percent was absorbed. These results indicate that there is no need to fear an overload of magnesium in the diet. Any excess will be excreted harmlessly, whereas a deficiency could have serious consequences.

Some researchers say that we don't absorb more because we evolved on a diet that was high in magnesium from foods such as greens, nuts, seeds, and grains and so didn't need mechanisms to conserve it. That could be one of the underlying reasons that we are so deficient—our diet has betrayed us.

A number of other conditions also influence the degree of absorption:

- Whether the intestines are healthy or diseased
- Availability of the protein transport molecule for magnesium
- Availability of parathyroid hormone
- The rate of water absorption, because magnesium is soluble in water
- The amounts of calcium, phosphorus, potassium,

sodium, and lactose (milk sugar) in the body, all of
which inhibit magnesium absorption

- Supplemental iron, which can impede magnesium
absorption and vice versa (if you take both, you
should take them several hours apart)

Whether the intestines are healthy or diseased is probably the
most important factor in magnesium absorption. Having written extensively on irritable bowel syndrome (IBS) and yeast
overgrowth in *IBS for Dummies* (coauthored with L. Christine
Wheeler, 2005) and *The Yeast Connection and Women's Health*
(coauthored with William G. Crook, 2005), I have great concern about magnesium absorption in people who have a leaky
gut—micropunctures caused by infection and injury to the intestinal lining that allow absorption of toxins into the bloodstream. The most common cause is overgrowth of the yeast
Candida albicans, which normally lives largely unnoticed in the
large intestine; when it moves into the small intestine, however, it sends out threadlike fibers that can create microscopic
holes in the intestinal tissue, causing what's called "leaky gut."
Yeast grows beyond its normal environment in the large intestine under the influence of antibiotics, cortisone and other
steroids, birth control pills, estrogen, and a high-sugar diet. It
produces up to 180 different by-products, most of which are
toxins that can be absorbed through a leaky gut.

Yeast toxins, inflammatory substances the body produces
as it tries to neutralize those toxins, and undigested food molecules all form barriers to the absorption of dietary and supplemental nutrients, including magnesium. I believe that IBS,
yeast overgrowth, and food allergies must all be addressed
in order to achieve optimal magnesium absorption. Reading
about these conditions, investigating the use of appropriate nutritional products, and consulting with appropriate and knowledgeable experts may be necessary in order to develop a strategy

these problems and ensure adequate magnesium
ption.

MAGNESIUM IS BLOCKED BY CERTAIN FOODS

It's important to know which foods are high or low in magnesium, but you should also know that certain foods contain
chemicals that block absorption of magnesium. For example,
there is much evidence that a high-protein diet only makes
magnesium deficiency worse, and if you are following such a
regimen, you should take at least 300 mg of supplemental
magnesium.[10] Another potential source of problems is the tan-
nin in tea, which binds and removes all minerals, including
magnesium, from the body. If you suspect you are magnesium
deficient, it's best to avoid both black and green tea, especially
if they are strongly bitter. Less bitter teas do not contain such
high amounts of tannins and may be less of a problem.

Oxalic acid, which is found in spinach and chard (among
other foods), and phytic acid, found in the hulls of seeds and
the bran of grains, can form insoluble compounds with magnesium and other minerals, causing them to be eliminated
rather than absorbed. Cooking vegetables removes most of the
oxalic acid, so steam spinach, chard, and other high-oxalic-
acid vegetables instead of eating or juicing them raw. Preventing the binding action of phytic acid in grains and seeds is not
so simple. Grains and seeds can be soaked for eight to twelve
hours to remove the phytic acid, but few people make this effort. A diet high in grains is another reason to take magnesium
supplements.

Soybeans, too, are high in phytic acid. Soy has one of the
highest phytate levels of any legume and, unlike others, its
phytic acid is not destroyed with extended cooking time. Only
fermentation (as is done in the production of miso and tem-

peh) will reduce the phytic acid levels of soy. This explains why I recommend only fermented soy and advise people to stay away from soy powders and soy milk as well as tofu, especially when these substitute for meat and dairy. As a cheap alternative to meat, soy (as soy protein isolate and textured vegetable protein) has exploded on the school lunch menu and in the fast-food industry. Too much soy can cause mineral deficiencies in children, who really need their minerals to build strong bones and teeth—the structures for adult health.

Moreover, menopausal women may be overusing soy (for its natural phytoestrogenic effects) and developing similar mineral deficiencies. While the phytoestrogens in soy may be helpful to older women, they are another reason to avoid using unfermented soy in the diets of growing boys and girls.

A JUNK-FOOD DIET LACKS MAGNESIUM

Even in a healthy diet with proper protein intake, the addition of 150 mg of elemental magnesium a day can make dramatic changes in health.[11] (See Chapter 18 for a full discussion of magnesium supplementation.) If even a good diet can leave you magnesium-deficient, a poor diet can seriously undermine your health.

We live in strange times, when people avidly watch gourmet-cooking shows while devouring junk food. Junk food provides 27 percent of most people's daily calories; an astounding 90 percent of our food dollar is spent on processed foods. People who drink soda and soft drinks may be magnesium-deficient because sugar uses up magnesium.[12, 13] Many carbonated beverages and processed foods (luncheon meats and hot dogs) contain phosphates, which bind with magnesium to make insoluble magnesium phosphate, which is not absorbed by the body.

DRUGS CAUSE MAGNESIUM DEFICIENCY

Ironically, one of the foremost magnesium experts, Mildred Seelig, M.D., began her research career in the 1960s working for drug companies. It was there she first noticed that many of the side effects of drugs were actually magnesium deficiency symptoms. It seemed to her that many drugs cause increased demand for and utilization of magnesium—for example, by creating acidity in the body, which then draws on available magnesium from the cells to try to neutralize the acid and minimize its toxic effects. Other drugs seemed to deplete magnesium from the body or, conversely, manifest their positive effects because they pulled magnesium from storage sites and increased the level of magnesium in the blood.[14]

The following commonly used drugs can create magnesium deficiencies:[15]

- Common diuretics (for high blood pressure)
- Bronchodilators, such as theophylline (for asthma)
- Birth control pills
- Insulin
- Digitalis (for some heart conditions)
- Tetracycline and certain other antibiotics
- Corticosteroids (for asthma)
- Cocaine
- Nicotine

DRUG INTERACTIONS WITH MAGNESIUM

Other drugs interact with magnesium in specific ways.[16] For example, magnesium is a muscle relaxant, so it enhances the actions of prescription muscle relaxants such as tubocurarine (used in surgery), barbiturates, hypnotics, and narcotics. These medications may be decreased under a doctor's supervision if you are on magnesium. In other words, you may not need as much muscle relaxant because magnesium is a natural relaxant. Tell your anesthesiologist before surgery if you are taking magnesium supplements.

Magnesium protects the kidneys, so supplementation may be beneficial during treatment with aminoglycoside antibiotics such as gentamicin and immunosuppressant drugs such as cyclosporin and cisplatin, which result in magnesium loss. Discuss this with your doctor.

Diuretics and cardiac drugs lower magnesium levels in the body. Diuretics throw off potassium, which is well known, but they also eliminate magnesium. Additional magnesium intake is recommended during administration of diuretics and cardiac glycosides such as digoxin. Check with your doctor.

Magnesium inhibits the absorption of iron, tetracycline, ciprofloxacin, vancomycin, isoniazid, chlorpromazine, trimethoprim, nitrofurantoin, and sodium fluoride. Take these medications two to three hours before or after magnesium supplements. (Sodium fluoride is prescribed for osteoporosis, although taking magnesium may be a wiser choice—especially since fluoride binds magnesium and makes it unavailable to the body. See Chapter 11 for more on osteoporosis.)

VITAMIN AND MINERAL INTERACTIONS WITH MAGNESIUM

Research has not yet progressed to the point where we know all the possible interactions of magnesium. Every year brings more intelligence on the subject.

- Both calcium and magnesium are required in order for either mineral to work properly.
- Sufficient vitamin D is necessary for the body to utilize magnesium.

- Magnesium enters into cells with the support of Vitamin B_1 (thiamine). If that water-soluble mineral is deficient, even if magnesium is absorbed, it won't get to its destination.
- Selenium helps magnesium stay inside cells where it belongs.

MAGNESIUM WASTING

There are genetic causes of magnesium wasting, where the kidneys just can't seem to hold on to this vital mineral, but they are very rare. And some people require high amounts of this mineral because most is lost through the kidneys. I was surprised when at a recent seminar a doctor came up and thanked me for my talk on magnesium and said he suffered from magnesium wasting. He reported that in spite of having a good diet, taking supplements, and being on no magnesium-wasting drugs such as diuretics or digitalis, he still had slightly high blood pressure, moderately high cholesterol, and leg cramping. When he read the first edition of *The Magnesium Miracle* he realized his problem might be magnesium deficiency. But even when he took more, he still had some symptoms. That's when he decided to do a magnesium challenge test (see Chapter 16) and found out he was not retaining much magnesium at all, even after an IV challenge.

The doctor began taking regular IV treatments of magnesium. As mentioned in Chapter 18, applying magnesium oil or gel helps people who need high amounts of magnesium avoid the expense and inconvenience of taking magnesium injections.

WHY HAVEN'T WE HEARD ABOUT MAGNESIUM?

The vast majority of us were not exposed to nutritional education in school. But what about doctors? As you may suspect, doctors generally do not learn about nutrition or nutrient supplementation in medical school because they are studying disease, not wellness. When you visit a medical doctor, you may think you are going there to improve your health or prevent illness, but doctors have little time to educate their patients about how to keep themselves well. And patients often will not change their lifestyle unless their doctor tells them to, believing that if vitamins were so important, the doctor would have told them to take supplements. (Of course, some patients don't change the way they live even when their doctor does tell them they have to lose weight and eat right.) However, nutrition is not even a medical specialty. It wasn't when I went to medical school in the 1970s and it still isn't today! That's why you won't hear most of the information I report in this book from your doctor—because it's outside his or her field.

WHEN ALL YOU HAVE IS A HAMMER

In the first two years of medical school I learned all about diseases; the second two years I studied drug treatments for those diseases. We spent no time on nutrient deficiencies. Have you heard the expression "When all you have is a hammer, everything begins to look like a nail"? That is very much the case with doctors and drug treatments. But even worse, with thousands of drugs in the pharmaceutical compendium, it is quite impossible for doctors to keep up on the latest drugs, and impossible to prevent side effects or serious drug interactions. Studies show that most doctors are unable to recognize drug interactions and confuse them with a need to increase the dose rather than stop the drug. Although allopathic (conventional) medicine is said to be scientific, most patients are on more than one drug at a time, and there are *no* studies proving the safety of drug combinations.

According to magnesium expert Mildred Seelig, M.D., while

a tremendous amount of magnesium research has been done in India, Britain, France, and other European countries, doctors in the United States use the excuse that not enough research has been done here for them to feel informed enough to prescribe it. Dr. Seelig calls this the "not-invented-here syndrome." Pioneers such as Drs. Bella and Burton Altura, however, continue to do original magnesium research in this country. Every year for the past forty years they have produced on average a dozen peer-reviewed journal articles on magnesium and ionic magnesium testing. Their research convinces even die-hard skeptics—when they take the time to become informed—of the clear need for magnesium supplementation and the absolute requirement for accurate testing.

DRUG COMPANIES FUND DRUG RESEARCH, NOT MINERAL RESEARCH

Medical science studies one symptom at a time, in isolation, and generally tries to find one cause for that symptom and one drug that treats it. The bias of medical research makes it search for a patentable drug that will eventually pay for the costly studies necessary to bring it to market. Everyone agrees that magnesium is indispensable for health, disease prevention, and all life processes, but it has been ignored because there is no profit to be made in selling a common nutrient. Magnesium cannot be patented, so pharmaceutical companies do not engage in magnesium research. There is no advertising budget for magnesium, compared to the hundreds of millions of dollars spent on advertising prescription drugs; nutrients do not get media attention. To make matters worse, over the past two decades the bulk of university funding has come from the pharmaceutical industry, which primarily funds drug research.[17] Scientific medicine ignores nutrient investigation in favor of drugs. Older research is also ignored by health providers. Doctors may have heard years ago that magnesium offered some promise in heart disease, but they haven't read any new studies, so they assume that the treatment must have not panned out.

Doctors seem to be waiting for a large clinical trial, for example, following twenty thousand people taking magnesium for life. It would have been nice if such a study had been initiated thirty years ago. Do we have the luxury of waiting for the results of such a study started now? No, we do not. Do we presently know enough about magnesium to recommend widespread supplementation? Yes, we do.

An analysis of seven major clinical studies shows that intravenous magnesium reduced the risk of death by 55 percent after acute heart attack. These results were published in the prestigious *British Medical Journal* and the widely read journal *Drugs.*[18, 19]

As noted, Drs. Bella and Burton Altura have been researching magnesium and its clinical application for over forty years.[20] The ionized magnesium electrode, produced by Nova Biomedical of Waltham, Massachusetts, at the Alturas' urging, and tested at the State University of New York's Downstate Medical Center, has given doctors a reliable magnesium test and taken the guesswork out of diagnosing magnesium deficiency.[21] With such testing in hundreds of clinical trials the Alturas have been able to show that as many as twenty-one varied health conditions are related to magnesium deficiency. These are the conditions listed on pages xviii–xxi and reported on in *The Magnesium Miracle.*

Dr. Alexander Mauskop, working with the Alturas, has proven the connection between migraines and magnesium many times over and puts magnesium treatment into practice at the New York Headache Center.[22, 23, 24] Dr. Mildred Seelig has contributed comprehensive reviews on magnesium at New York Medical College, the American College of Nutrition, and more recently at the Department of Nutrition, University of North Carolina.[25, 26] Dr. Jean Durlach, president of the International Society for the Development of Research on Magnesium (SDRM), editor in chief of *Magnesium Research*, and professor at St. Vincent de Paul Hospital in Paris, has done extensive reviews of ongoing magnesium research.[27, 28]

All these magnesium experts agree that we must no longer sit on the sidelines or reserve judgment on the benefits of magnesium; we need to implement what we know, *now.*

PART TWO

MAGNESIUM-DEFICIENT CONDITIONS

═══

CHAPTER THREE

ANXIETY AND DEPRESSION

THREE THINGS YOU NEED TO KNOW ABOUT MAGNESIUM, ANXIETY, AND DEPRESSION

1. Magnesium deficiency can produce symptoms of anxiety or depression, including muscle weakness, fatigue, eye twitches, insomnia, anorexia, apathy, apprehension, poor memory, confusion, anger, nervousness, and rapid pulse.
2. Serotonin, the "feel-good" brain chemical that is boosted by Prozac, depends on magnesium for its production and function.
3. Magnesium supports our adrenal glands, which are overworked by stress.

Each year millions of people are introduced to the merry-go-round of psychiatric drugs and psychological counseling for symptoms that may in fact be rooted in magnesium deficiency. Additional millions try unsuccessfully to cope with their problems by turning to overeating, cigarettes, alcohol, street drugs, and other addictive behavior to suppress their pain. We are a nation suffering a 32 percent incidence of anxiety, depression, and drug problems. Social epidemiologist Myrna Weissman at Columbia University reports that more and more Americans are becoming depressed, getting depressed at a younger age, and experiencing more severe and frequent periods of depression. Each generation born in the twentieth century has suffered more depression than the previous one, and since World War II the overall rate of depression has more than doubled.[1, 2] A recent study in the *Archives of General Psychiatry* showed a doubling of depression in women from 1970 to 1992, with the use of psychiatric drugs skyrocketing as a result.[3]

People do not get anxiety, panic attacks, or depression because they have a deficiency of Valium or Prozac. Our bodies do not require these substances for essential metabolic processes. However, we can develop a myriad of psychological symptoms because of a deficiency of magnesium, a nutrient our bodies do require. Does it make any sense to merely switch our addictions from sugar, alcohol, drugs, and cigarettes to prescription medication without looking at the possible underlying metabolic causes? Psychiatrists all too often rely on prescription drugs for suffering patients and have no insight into the metabolic functioning of the mind and body and what happens when nutrients are deficient. Anxiety and depression are often nutrient-deficiency diseases and chemical sensitivities, certainly *not* drug-deficiency diseases.

A remarkable study of almost 500 depressed people by Drs. Cox and Shealy found that the majority of sufferers were magnesium-deficient. The authors of the study advised clinicians that they should consider the distinct possibility of a therapeutic benefit from the use of magnesium therapy in chronic depression.[4]

ADRENALINE WASTES MAGNESIUM

It's not just a theory that stress causes magnesium deficiency and a lack of magnesium magnifies stress. Experiments where adrenaline is given intravenously produce a decrease in magnesium as well as calcium, potassium, and sodium. Without enough magnesium to relax arteries and muscles, blood pressure rises and the heart muscle cramps. When the IV adrenaline is stopped, the body recovers in about thirty minutes and potassium rises. However, it takes much longer for magnesium to reach normal levels.

There are over a dozen major metabolic processes that are affected by adrenaline, including heart rate, blood pressure, blood vessel constriction, and muscular contraction. Each of these functions requires magnesium and leads to wasting of this important mineral if the symptoms continue.

Darcy had driven across a mile-long bridge every day for years, so why one morning did she suddenly feel as though she would die if she didn't pull over? She was sweating and her heart was pounding; she felt sick to her stomach and couldn't get her breath. What was happening to her? Fortunately, she had her cell phone and called her best friend, Sara, who helped her calm herself and make her way across the bridge safely. Later, while talking with Sara to try to make sense of the episode, Darcy said she had been on a liquid protein diet for a few weeks. Sara pointed out that it could have thrown something out of balance, and she reminded Darcy that she had warned her of the dangers of this type of diet.

The two women reviewed the list of supplements that Darcy had been taking as part of the program and found that she had neglected to take the magnesium that had been suggested. Sara grabbed a natural health encyclopedia and, sure enough, magnesium deficiency was listed as one of the possible causes of panic attacks.

If Sara had read further, she would have found that the body demands more magnesium when on a liquid protein diet and that the dangers of such a diet have been documented for decades.[5] By eating only protein, Darcy had set herself up for a terrifying attack. Fortunately, she discovered this before pursuing a prescription for a tranquilizer to deal with the frightening symptoms of panic attack.

Lack of magnesium may not have been the only cause of Darcy's panic attack. As well as creating an extra demand for magnesium, her high-protein diet could have led to symptoms of hypoglycemia. When blood sugar (glucose) is low, the body reacts with a surge of adrenaline to bring glucose levels back to normal in order to keep this essential nutrient fueling the brain. Adrenaline acts to speed the heart and retrieve glucose from liver storage. Sometimes people perceive a normal adrenaline rush as a panic attack. Interestingly enough, magnesium is also a requirement for proper blood sugar control.

Women tend to pay attention to their feelings and interpret symptoms such as panic attacks as signs of emotional imbalance, for which they seek support. The support they get, however, is often in the form of a prescription for an antianxiety drug instead of sound advice to eat a better diet, exercise, and take the right balance of supplements.

Magnesium deficiency can be an underlying cause of anxiety and depression, as determined in several clinical trials.[6] Symptoms of chronic magnesium deficiency include anxious behavior, hyperemotionality, apathy, apprehension, poor memory, confusion, anger, nervousness, muscle weakness, fatigue, headaches, insomnia, light-headedness, dizziness, nervous fits, the feeling of a lump in the throat, impaired breathing, muscle cramps (including leg cramps), a tingling or pricking or creeping feeling on the skin, rapid pulse, chest pain, palpitations, and abnormal heart rhythm.[7, 8] See the list of 100 possible symptoms and factors indicating magnesium deficiency on pages 17–20.

Even the hyperventilation that may accompany anxiety can further drop magnesium levels. Why is this? Hyperventilation makes the blood more alkaline, which must be neutralized with an intricate dance of sodium, potassium, calcium, and magnesium. It's much more unobtrusive, however, to take magnesium supplements for anxiety than to pull out a paper bag and breathe into it.

An important study in 1995 showed that even marginal magnesium deficiency could induce the brain to become hyperexcitable, as shown by EEG measurements. The study lasted six months, with thirteen women ingesting a total of 115 milligrams of magnesium daily, only 30 percent of the RDA, for the first three months, during which time their EEGs showed hyperexcitability. During the second three months, they received 315 mg daily—a little closer to the 360 mg RDA recommended for women. However, even on this low dose of magnesium (315 mg), it took only six weeks for EEG readings to show significant improvement in brain function and decreased excitability.[9]

ANXIETY

Stress is so prevalent in our daily life that we have become desensitized to it and the message it is trying to give us, which is to slow down. Anxiety is a chemical reaction created when the adrenal glands respond to a stressful event, such as low blood sugar, by releasing adrenaline. Adrenaline is very useful if you're trying to escape from a dangerous situation, because it stimulates the fight-or-flight response: the heart starts pumping faster; digestion slows down; energy stores are released from the liver and made available to the heart, lungs, and muscles; and the muscles of the arms and legs are activated. All of these responses require magnesium. So each time we experience any kind of stress, our magnesium stores are tapped to create energy. This magnesium depletion itself stresses the body, which can result in panic attacks, which equals yet more stress. Not only do our overworked adrenals cause magnesium depletion, but even more adrenaline is released under stress when magnesium levels are low in the body, leaving people feeling irritable, nervous, edgy, or even ready to explode. It's the proverbial Catch-22.[10] To put an end to anxiety, magnesium needs to be replaced.

During stress reactions, calcium is also required to stimulate the release of adrenaline, but calcium excess causes a flood of adrenaline. However, having sufficient magnesium will buffer excess calcium and keep it within normal levels, limiting the stress response. Magnesium is important because it naturally diminishes the excitability of the nervous system and lowers the level of calcium around nerve cells. This function of magnesium is also significant in heart disease and other stress-induced illness.[11, 12]

CHRONIC STRESS

According to Hans Selye, the Canadian doctor famous for his work on stress in the 1960s, magnesium is also depleted when the body shifts from a short-term fight-or-flight reaction to a chronic stress reaction. The adrenal glands produce cortisol, a type of cortisone, and another stress hormone, norepinephrine, which acts like adrenaline and also causes magnesium depletion.

Chronic stress can come from feeling insecure and threatened, or from exposure to toxic chemicals, heavy metals, or even loud noise, all of which assault the nervous system and overwork the immune system. For example, constant loud noise in an industrial work setting induced a significant increase of serum magnesium (as magnesium was released from tissues) and significantly increased urinary excretion of magnesium, indicating a magnesium deficiency, which lasted for forty-eight hours after exposure.[13]

MAGNESIUM AND MUSICIANS

One case of sound-induced magnesium deficiency became evident to a parent who heard me talking about this condition on a New York radio station. She called in to the program and said that a few months after her son began playing in a rock band his left eyelid started to twitch uncontrollably. Listening to me on the radio show, she realized that it might be due to magnesium deficiency. Her son's twitching was likely a result of magnesium being used to buffer against the stress of sounds at a decibel level that sets off alarm bells in the body. Loud sounds cause a reflexive fight-or-flight response, and constant loud sound is not something the body gets used to and ignores—it must continually adapt to the noise, all the while using up valuable nutrients such as magnesium to do that job.

Exposure to loud music can increase urinary excretion of magnesium, which lasts for days after exposure. If magnesium is not replaced through an excellent diet and supplements, magnesium deficiency symptoms such as the 100 listed on pages 17–20 may begin to appear. Although I do know some rock musicians who are vegetarians and don't smoke or drink alcohol, they may not be the norm. Smoking, coffee, alcohol, and the rock star lifestyle all contribute to magnesium deficiency.

Musicians have more than one reason to use magnesium. Nervousness, anticipation, and anxiety are all part of the buildup to a musical performance, whether it's classical, rock, punk, or rap. To deal with the anxiety and the resulting elevated heart rate that often accompanies it, musicians may feel they have to turn to drugs, alcohol, or even medication. Inderal (propranolol) is a beta-blocker that is normally prescribed to treat high blood pressure and heart arrhythmias. However, it's also called "the musicians' underground drug" because it is used for performance anxiety. It's underground in the sense that it's not widely spoken about and also because anxiety is an off-label use of Inderal, which means that the FDA has not approved the drug for this use. However, there have been some small studies reporting that musicians felt better about their performance on beta-blockers.

What does Inderal do that makes it so attractive to musicians? Beta-blockers such as Inderal block physical reactions to fear. When your heart begins to race, your palms start to sweat, and you just want to run as fast and as far as you can, this describes the fight-or-flight response. Adrenaline is pumped from the adrenal glands to ready your muscles to run or fight. But what musicians need is to be calm, so that their hands don't slip off their instrument from shaking and sweating. They need their heart to stop thumping so loudly in their head that they can't hear their cue or even see the conductor or band leader. And for band leaders or conductors, the fear inherent in being responsible for the success of the performance is heightened even further.

Beta-blockers are used to decrease heart rate, but some of them, including Inderal, also cause constriction of the bronchial tubes, which makes them dangerous to use if you have asthma. They can also worsen congestive heart failure, diabetes, allergic reactions, and Raynaud's syndrome. Some people may have no side effects using small doses only on rare occasions, but higher doses and becoming physically dependent on beta-blockers to calm you before every performance can take its toll.

Inderal is contraindicated in pregnancy and has the following side effects.

MOST FREQUENT
Decreased sexual function, drowsiness, fatigue, general weakness, insomnia

LESS FREQUENT
Abdominal pain with cramps, anxiety, bronchospastic pulmonary disease, chronic heart failure, constipation, depression, diarrhea, dizziness, nasal congestion, nausea, nervousness, sensation of cold, vomiting

RARE
Agranulocytosis, allergic reactions, anaphylaxis, arthralgia, back pain, chest pain, conduction disorder of the heart, dry eye, dysgeusia, erythema, erythema multiforme, exfoliative dermatitis, hallucinations, impaired cognition, laryngismus, leukopenia, nightmares, ocular irritation, orthostatic hypotension, pharyngitis, pruritus of skin, psoriasiform eruption, severe dyspnea, Stevens-Johnson syndrome, thrombocytopenic disorder, toxic epidermal necrolysis

Most musicians may not know all the side effects of Inderal; they take the medication because they need to, and they know lots of others who are doing the same. They may not realize that their sexual dysfunction, insomnia, and skin rash are due to the medication or that the medication removes the edge that adrenaline gives them. And for some, even if they do know, it's the price they pay in order to function in their profession. What they don't know is how much more effective and safe magnesium is for anxiety and stress. It can also function to increase energy and performance levels that Inderal may actually block. The absolute irony of using Inderal for anxiety is that it is known to reduce the levels of magnesium in the body, causing increased excretion through the urine. So if magnesium depletion is a cause of your anxiety, Inderal can make it worse. Another benefit of taking magnesium is reduction in the buildup of lactic acid that occurs after hours of playing. Repetitive motion injuries common to musicians can be eased by taking magnesium orally, using magnesium oil or gel on the injured arm or shoulder, and using homeopathic magnesium as needed. (See page 253 for more on homeopathic magnesium.)

The best oral form of magnesium for musicians is magnesium glycinate, two 200 mg tablets per day with an extra one or two on the day of a performance. Other enhancements to performance include a good balanced diet to overcome any symptoms of hypoglycemia, which also causes anxiety; meditation and relaxation therapies; and yoga, swimming, walking, and other forms of exercise to increase circulation and burn off excess adrenaline. It is inadvisable to suddenly stop using Inderal if you have been taking it regularly; check with your doctor about weaning off it as you increase your doses of magnesium and see the benefits.

MAGNESIUM-DEFICIENT KIDS

No, it's not just adults who can get anxious because of magnesium-deficient diets. Our children are also susceptible when their favorite foods are magnesium-deficient hot dogs, pizza, and soda. The stress in their lives—from peer pressure, academic and athletic performance pressures, worries about body image, the changes and hormonal fluctuations of puberty, exposure to negative events and violence through the media—also contributes. Even playing in a band can be a risk factor! Children are underdiagnosed when it comes to magnesium deficiency, but they can have magnesium deficiencies for the same reasons as adults. Attention deficit hyperactivity disorder (ADHD), autism, juvenile delinquency, and childhood depression are associated with magnesium deficiency, and some say these conditions can be caused by it.[14]

Dr. Sharna Olfman, a professor of clinical and developmental psychology, issues the following warning in her book *No Child Left Different:*

> The number of American children being diagnosed with psychiatric illnesses has soared over the past decade and a half. The National Institute of Mental Health (NIMH) estimates that today, one in ten children and adolescents in the United States "suffers from mental illness severe enough to result in significant functional impairment." During this same time period, psychotropic drugs have become the treatment of first choice rather than the treatment of last resort. Recent years have witnessed a threefold increase in the use of psychotropic medication among patients under twenty years of age, and prescriptions for preschoolers have been skyrocketing. Over 10 million children and adolescents are currently on antidepressants, and about 5 million children are taking stimulant medications such as Ritalin.[15]

In 2005, Columbia University initiated a program called Teen Screen throughout forty states, which screened teens and children for mental health problems. Unfortunately, such screening usually leads to the prescribing of more drugs. Instead of reaching for Ritalin or Prozac for kids, consider whether they're getting enough magnesium first. In fact, if these children were simply taken off sugar and put on magnesium, we would have much happier children and thus far fewer side effects from powerful drugs.

Dr. Leo Galland, author of *Superimmunity for Kids,* speculates that hyperactive children need extra magnesium due to their constantly high adrenaline levels. Dr. Galland recommends 6 mg per pound of weight per day (for example, 240 mg for a 40-lb child). Because magnesium is hard to find in a form suitable for young children, he suggests 1 tbsp of magnesium citrate a day or 1½ tsp of milk of magnesia a day. These are both laxatives in much larger doses, but in such small doses they supply the necessary magnesium without a laxative effect.[16] If there is any concern about a laxative effect, have your child take several smaller doses of magnesium citrate a day and not take it all in one dose.

SEROTONIN, MAGNESIUM, AND DEPRESSION

You may be familiar with serotonin, the body's natural "feel-good" brain chemical. Magnesium is important in the serotonin story because it is a necessary element in the release and uptake of serotonin by brain cells. With proper amounts of magnesium, nature makes sufficient serotonin and you experience emotional balance. But when stress depletes magnesium, a vicious cycle spins out of control, and depression can occur. The body needs magnesium in order to release and bind adequate amounts of serotonin in the brain for balanced mental functioning.

The pharmaceutical industry has focused its research for the treatment of depression on selective serotonin reuptake inhibitors (SSRIs), such as Prozac, to capitalize on serotonin's chemical effects instead of giving serotonin what it really needs—magnesium. SSRIs create artificially elevated levels of serotonin in the body by preventing its breakdown and elimination; serotonin lingers longer in the brain and theoretically causes mood elevation. This is what is *supposed* to happen, but everyone has a different reaction to the manipulation of their brain chemicals. For some people, prolonged, rising levels of serotonin can liberate them from a long depression. For others, the drug can lead to anxiety and irritability. A small but significant group can feel released from their apathy and act on suicidal or homicidal thoughts. Another group of people tend to have flattened moods in which they can neither weep nor laugh, keeping them from the extremes of depression or mania but relegating them to a one-dimensional life.

This was Maggie's situation. She was on Prozac and desperately trying to come off it because she was unable to cry or experience real emotions. Maggie was down to one-quarter of a 10 mg tablet but was afraid to stop in case her depression came back. She also had high blood pressure, high cholesterol, periodic muscle cramps, and constipation. I asked her to have her magnesium tested, and her cardiologist said it was normal; he said she didn't need magnesium but should continue to take her five prescription medications to control her symptoms. She called me when her GP thought her worsening muscle cramps were a major blood clot in the leg. We didn't have time to ship a blood sample to the lab that performs red blood cell magnesium testing, so I encouraged her to take 300 mg of magnesium twice a day and go for a Doppler scan to rule out blood clots. Fortunately, the scan was negative, so Maggie was able to avoid several more medications to treat blood clots, and the magnesium was already working to relieve her symptoms. Within a few weeks Maggie was finally off the last small amount of Prozac and able to laugh and cry again.

TREATMENT FOR ANXIETY AND DEPRESSION

DIET

Avoid food additives, artificial sweeteners, sugar, and wheat. Eat a whole-foods diet—organic, if possible—and avoid processed and junk food. Also read *The Yeast Connection and Women's Health* (Crook and Dean, 2005) and *IBS for Dummies* (Dean and Wheeler, 2005) since both yeast and IBS are associated with anxiety and depression. Understanding and treating these conditions under the supervision of a knowledgeable practitioner can enhance use of the following supplements.

SUPPLEMENTS

Magnesium citrate: 300 mg twice a day

Calcium citrate: 500 mg daily

B complex: 50–100 mg per day (derived in whole or in part from natural food sources)

5-hydroxytryptamine (5-HTP): 50–100 mg half an hour before meals, three times a day (this is an amino acid that crosses the blood-brain barrier and is naturally converted into serotonin; it has the same action as Prozac but no side effects)

St. John's wort: 300 mg standardized extract three times a day

SLEEP AIDS

Melatonin: 2–3 mg one hour before bedtime

5-hydroxytryptamine (5-HTP): 50–200 mg half an hour before bedtime, on an empty stomach

Hops, valerian, and skullcap herbal combinations: one or two 500 mg capsules before bedtime

STRESS RELEASE

Exercise is excellent for treating both anxiety and depression (try yoga, walking, biking, Pilates, T-Tapp, and swimming), as are prayer, meditation, long baths, journal writing, and Emotional Freedom Techniques (EFT).

Because depression can be so debilitating, even life-threatening, it's understandable that doctors feel strong measures are required to combat it, but these strong measures don't always work. The alternative that many doctors are missing is the nutrient connection. Magnesium deficiency is a potential cause for every type of depression. All treatment protocols should begin with adequate doses of this valuable mineral.[17]

═══

CHAPTER FOUR

MIGRAINES AND PAIN

THREE THINGS YOU NEED TO KNOW ABOUT MAGNESIUM AND MIGRAINES

1. Magnesium prevents platelet aggregation, which helps to avoid the thickened blood and tiny clots that can cause blood vessel spasms and the pain of a migraine.
2. Magnesium relaxes the head and neck muscle tension that makes migraines worse.
3. Magnesium, vitamin B_2, and the herb feverfew are an important migraine treatment combination.

Martha knew that a migraine was looming when the sparks and wavy lines appeared before her eyes. Working became impossible, and she knew she would be looking at the loss of at least one day to a severe migraine attack. Medications such as codeine and ergotamine had not helped her over the years, instead making her feel drugged and tired after the headache finally passed. And the fancy new drugs Imitrex, Depakote, and Midrin did nothing for her head pain but did give her chest pain and make her more sick to her stomach. All Martha could do was lie in a darkened room with a cool cloth over her eyes, too nauseated to eat. This time, however, instead of trying to keep hydrated with lots of diet soda, as she usually did, she was going to drink mineral water with lemon and natural fruit juice.

Martha's daughter Mary, a nurse, had told her that aspartame, the sweetener in diet soda, causes headaches. Even though Martha loved her diet pop—she suspected that she was addicted to it, drinking two liters a day on average—she knew she had to do something to stop these headaches, both the daily ones and the one or two migraines a week.

Over the next few days, Martha's skin itched and she was nauseated, dizzy, and depressed. She thought she was having a reaction to the medication she had taken for her migraine, but Mary told her she was going through aspartame withdrawal. She was also having strong cravings for her diet soda, but Mary insisted that she stay off it. Mary did some more research on aspartame and how to cope with withdrawal and brought her mother a bottle of magnesium citrate supplements. The 150 mg three times a day seemed to help right away. By the next week, Martha's head felt clearer; she was more alert and less achy. She hadn't even realized that her joints and muscles had been tight and sore until she no longer had those symptoms. To her great relief, two weeks after eliminating aspartame from her diet, she realized that she hadn't had one of those headaches that she used to get daily. After two months of strictly avoiding aspartame, she still had no more headaches or migraines, except once after she had eaten something she had not known contained artificial sweetener. That convinced her even more that, for her, aspartame was poison.

ASPARTAME AND MSG: EXCITOTOXINS

Aspartame is, in fact, an excitotoxin, one of a group of substances, usually acidic amino acids, that in high amounts react with specialized receptors in the brain, causing destruction of certain types of neurons.

A growing number of neurosurgeons and neurologists are convinced that excitotoxins play a critical role in the development of several neurological disorders, including migraines, seizures, learning disorders in children, and neurodegenerative disorders such as Alzheimer's disease, Parkinson's disease, Huntington's disease, and amyotrophic lateral sclerosis (ALS).[1] Glutamate and aspartate are two powerful amino acids that act as neurotransmitters in the brain in very small concentrations, but they are also commonly available in food additives. Glutamate is in MSG, a flavor enhancer, and in hydrolyzed vegetable protein, found in hundreds of processed foods. Aspartate is one of three components of aspartame (NutraSweet, Equal), a sugar substitute. In higher concentrations as food additives, these chemicals constantly stimulate brain cells and can cause them to undergo a process of cell death known as excitotoxicity—the cells are excited to death.

HYPOGLYCEMIA

The brain becomes extremely vulnerable to excitotoxins during episodes of low blood sugar or hypoglycemia. Pound for pound, the brain uses more blood sugar than any other part of the body. Low blood sugar occurs when you are malnourished or even when you skip meals. It also occurs in individuals whose adrenal glands are depleted and can't mount the necessary adrenaline response to raise blood sugar when it gets too low. Magnesium is responsible for balancing blood sugar. With sufficient magnesium and balanced meals to prevent low blood sugar, you can protect yourself against headaches, attention deficit hyperactivity disorder, mood disorders, and even premenstrual tension. Supporting the brain as much as possible with safe nutrients and a safe environment, you may never need the brain-altering medications that are prescribed for these disorders.

Medically, hypoglycemia occurs when blood sugar (glucose) drops to a low of 50 mg/dl (normal is about 80–110 mg/dl). If you eat a highly refined diet with lots of white sugar and white flour, foods whose carbohydrates are rapidly absorbed into the bloodstream, your blood sugar will quickly become elevated; when it reaches a certain maximum, insulin enters the bloodstream and quickly ushers the excess glucose into the cells of the body, causing your blood sugar to drop. The more sugar you eat and absorb, the more insulin is released and the quicker your blood sugar can fall. This abrupt drop causes adrenaline to be released from the adrenal glands to make sure that the blood sugar does not fall so low that you faint. When that adrenaline mobilizes the sugar stores in the liver to elevate your blood sugar, however, it also produces a fight-or-flight reaction, which may give you a sense of anxiety or impending doom. It may even feel like a panic attack because you don't equate your symptoms with low blood sugar. At this point, if you eat something to pick you up or comfort you, such as a candy bar or an aspartame-containing diet drink, or if you are exposed to other environmental toxins, your glucose-deprived, magnesium-deficient brain will be more vulnerable to the effects of the excitotoxins. Many diseases of the nervous system are being associated with excitotoxin buildup in the brain, including migraines, seizures, strokes, and brain injury.

If you have magnesium deficiency and regularly use aspartame, the toxicity is magnified and can result in headaches and migraines. You can easily identify whether your headaches are caused by aspartame: give yourself sixty days without any aspartame and judge for yourself. And if you want to minimize the withdrawal effects, take 150 mg of elemental magnesium three or four times a day (see page 243 for more on dosages).

Magnesium helps prevent the chain of events that causes cell death due to low blood sugar and exposure to other toxins besides excitotoxins. One of the most important neuroprotectants known, magnesium helps defend our cells against potential neurotoxins in our environment, such as pesticides, herbicides, food additives, solvents, and cleaning products.[2] Drs. Michael and Mary Dan Eades, authors of *Protein Power*, state that if they had only one supplement to give their patients, they would choose magnesium above all others.[3] In Chapter 13 we will talk more about the myriad toxins to which we are subjected on a daily basis, how we can avoid them, and how magnesium can protect us from harm.

MIGRAINE MECHANISMS

Twenty-five million Americans suffer from migraines. Statistically, women have more migraines than men, especially in the twenty-to-fifty-year age group. The following biochemical events involving low magnesium have been identified in migraine sufferers and may set the stage for a migraine attack.[4]

- In nonmenopausal women, estrogen rises before the period, causing a shift of blood magnesium into bone and muscles. As a result, magnesium levels in the brain are lowered.
- When magnesium is low, it is unable to do its job to counteract the clotting action of calcium on the blood. Tiny blood clots are said to clog up tiny brain blood vessels, leading to migraines. Several other substances

that help create blood clots are increased when magnesium is too low.
- Low brain magnesium promotes neurotransmitter hyperactivity and nerve excitation that can lead to headaches.

Several conditions that trigger migraines are also associated with magnesium deficiency, including pregnancy, alcohol intake, usage of some diuretic drugs, stress, and menstruation. Magnesium deficiency is related to migraines in so many ways.

- Magnesium relaxes blood vessels and allows them to dilate, reducing the spasms and constrictions that can cause migraines.
- Magnesium regulates the action of brain neurotransmitters and inflammatory substances, which may play a role in migraines when unbalanced.
- Magnesium inhibits excess platelet aggregation, preventing the formation of tiny clots that can block blood vessels and cause pain.
- Magnesium relaxes muscles and prevents the buildup of lactic acid, which, along with muscle tension, can worsen head pain.

A group of 3,000 patients given 200 mg of magnesium daily had an 80 percent reduction in their migraine symptoms.[5] This study did not have a control group, so the results could be questioned, but it aroused a great deal of excitement and triggered a flurry of research on magnesium and migraines. Much of that research was done by Dr. Alexander Mauskop, director of the New York Headache Center, working with Drs. Bella and Burton Altura, who have been studying migraines and migraine treatments for about ten years. Their research team consistently found that magnesium is deficient in people with migraine and many other types of headache and, even more important, that treating the deficiency alleviates the headache.

Dr. Mauskop with the Drs. Altura undertook many research studies using sensitive magnesium ion electrodes.[6] During one of the first studies they found a deficiency in magnesium ions but not serum magnesium in migraine patients.[7] This discrepancy shows the lack of correlation between magnesium-deficient states and serum magnesium. This is because only 1 percent of the magnesium in the body is found in the blood (serum). A measurement of magnesium ions, the actual working magnesium, is much closer to the total amount of magnesium in the body.

When migraine sufferers with low magnesium ion levels were given intravenous magnesium, they experienced a complete alleviation of their symptoms, including sensitivity to light and sound.[8] Subsequent studies of migraine patients confirmed a common pattern and support a role for magnesium deficiency in the development of headaches.[9] The researchers found that infusion of magnesium resulted in a rapid and sustained relief of acute migraine. Because of an excellent safety profile and low cost, they recommend oral magnesium supplementation for migraine sufferers at a level of 6 mg/kg/day.[10]

Patients with cluster headaches, a very severe form of recurrent headache, have also been reported to have low magnesium ion levels. Some people suffer up to twenty bouts of pain daily in a siege that can last for months. Another study from Altura, Altura, and Mauskop examined the possibility that patients with cluster headaches and low magnesium ion levels may respond to an intravenous infusion of magnesium sulfate. Within fifteen minutes of an intravenous dose of magnesium, nine patients with cluster headaches had their acute headache aborted.[11] Blood ionized magnesium testing thus proves to be useful in elucidating the cause of cluster headaches and in identifying patients who may benefit from treatment with magnesium, much as it does for migraines.[12]

Another research team treated eighty-one patients who suffered ongoing migraine headaches with 300 mg of magnesium twice a day. The frequency of migraines was reduced by 41.6 percent in the magnesium group but by only 15.8 percent in a control group that received placebos. The number of migraine days and drug consumption for pain also decreased significantly in the magnesium group. High-dose oral magnesium appears to be effective in migraine treatment and prevention.[13]

SUPPLEMENTS FOR MIGRAINE

Identify food allergies that may trigger migraines
Magnesium citrate: 300 mg two or three times per day
Calcium citrate: 500 mg once per day
Vitamin B$_2$ (riboflavin): 400 mg per day
Vitamin B complex: 50 mg per day (it is necessary to take the complex to prevent imbalances if you are taking large amounts of one B vitamin)
Feverfew (*Tanacetum parthenium*): 100 mg per day
Stress therapies
Regular exercise
Aspirin has been used to treat headaches for decades. Magnesium-buffered aspirin, however, is preferred by heavy users. Could magnesium be responsible for some of its beneficial effects? The same question applies to buffered aspirin used in heart disease

---

In Dr. Mauskop's *What Your Doctor May Not Tell You About Migraines* he outlines his "triple therapy" for migraines. It includes magnesium, vitamin B$_2$ (riboflavin), and a well-known migraine herb, feverfew.

MUSCLE PAIN AND SPASMS

A patient came for a consultation and wanted a total body X-ray because she was having such severe episodes of pain—her whole body would go into spasm—that she thought she must have cancer. I asked her to try taking 300 mg of magnesium three times a day. Within three days she no longer had the spasms, and after three weeks she was free of pain.

THREE THINGS YOU NEED TO KNOW
ABOUT MAGNESIUM AND MUSCLE PAIN

1. Magnesium helps muscles relax.
2. Magnesium eliminates spasms.
3. Magnesium relaxes blood vessels in the fingers to treat Raynaud's syndrome.

Although this patient did not have cancer, research has shown that even the pain of cancer can respond to magnesium. Cancer sometimes metastasizes into nerve bundles located in the neck or lower back and may not respond to even the strongest analgesics such as morphine. There is a special receptor site called NMDA that is responsible for creating this type of nerve pain; magnesium helps block this receptor. In cases of severe pain, intravenous magnesium has shown very powerful analgesic effects.[14]

Muscle twitches, tics, and spasms may seem like minor irritations to the onlooker, but to the person suffering, it's like water torture—only instead of water slowly dripping on your forehead, your eye or lip or a small muscle in your leg may constantly jump and writhe. Muscle twitches are a sure sign of magnesium deficiency. The nervous system is hyperexcitable and fires off small muscle groups to try to release some tension. But the only way to eliminate muscle spasms and twitches is by relaxing the nervous system with the proper amounts of magnesium.

RAYNAUD'S SYNDROME

Sally had terrible leg cramps. During the night, her legs felt jumpy and twitchy and kept her awake. If she did fall asleep, muscle cramps in her calf would wake her up. In addition, her fingers began turning white, blue, or red at different times. A young internist diagnosed her as having Raynaud's syndrome, a circulatory condition caused by the spasm of tiny arteries, especially in the hands and feet.

Raynaud's syndrome may occur suddenly or as a result of other chronic illnesses such as connective tissue disease, trauma, or pulmonary hypertension, in which cases it is called Raynaud's phenomenon. Raynaud's syndrome is seen mostly in young women and rarely leads to damage of the extremities. Cold is often the only stimulus that initiates the blood vessel spasms, which may last from minutes to hours. Emotional stress can also play a role in bringing on an attack. Besides the noted color changes there can be agonizing pain, especially when the fingers are rewarming. Symptoms of tingling, numbness, and burning are common. Many people who have this condition just put up with it. Even if they consult their doctors for a diagnosis, there is no safe, effective drug treatment for it (sometimes calcium channel blockers are used).

Fortunately, Sally's internist knew that magnesium is the most effective treatment for both muscle cramps and Raynaud's because it improves circulation, stops spasms, and minimizes stress reactions. He put her on magnesium, 300 mg twice a day, and a daily multiple vitamin and mineral; after two months he added calcium, 500 mg twice a day.

It took three months for the Raynaud's to respond, but Sally couldn't believe how much better she felt in the meantime. The muscle cramps improved within a week, and symptoms that she had thought were just part of getting old dramatically improved. Her energy increased, as she was able to sleep better. Her bowel movements were also more regular, and she was much calmer than she had been in a long time.

Nutritional recommendations for Raynaud's include liver-cleansing foods such as beets, dandelion greens, burdock root, and lemons, and foods rich in magnesium, including nuts, seeds, green vegetables, and whole grains. Foods to avoid or reduce to lessen the symptoms of Raynaud's syndrome include meat, alcohol, spices, and fatty, rich, fried, or salty foods.

SUPPLEMENTS FOR RAYNAUD'S

Magnesium citrate: 300 mg twice per day
Calcium citrate: 500 mg per day
Vitamin E as mixed tocopherols: 800 IU per day
Evening primrose oil: 6 capsules per day
Vitamin B_3: 100 mg three times a day (this vitamin sometimes causes the body to flush, as it increases circulation to the extremities)
Quercetin (a bioflavonoid): 500 mg per day

TOURETTE SYNDROME

Tourette syndrome was first defined in 1885 by a French physician. It is characterized by violent muscle contortions called motor tics and vocal disruptions combined with outbursts of swearing or obscenities. The vocal tics occur in only 5–15 percent of patients. Tourette syndrome itself was thought to be a rare condition; however, the National Institutes of Health report that the prevalence of Tourette syndrome is substantially higher than previously estimated.[15]

The NIH also reports that Tourette syndrome is associated with obsessive-compulsive disorder, ADHD, and learning problems in children who also have tics and rage attacks. A gene or genes responsible for Tourette syndrome have yet to be found.

The muscle contortions that characterize Tourette syndrome are increased by stress and associated with anxiety, depression, and sleep disorders. Since all these associated conditions are affected by magnesium, it only makes sense to look at magnesium deficiency as a possible cause. Research has defined the central role of magnesium deficiency in Tourette syndrome, and this bears further investigation.[16]

MAGNESIUM AND EXERCISE

When your muscles are engaged in the rapid-fire contraction and relaxation of physical exercise, if there is too much calcium (the initiator of contractions) and too little magnesium (the initiator of relaxation), muscle cramps and a buildup of lactic acid can result. Even though most athletes and coaches don't know it, magnesium is one of the most important nutrients athletes can possibly take.

As noted earlier, cells use energy packets called ATP (adenosine triphosphate), which are formed under the influence of magnesium. Some of the first studies showing the relationship between magnesium and physical performance were done on animals and found that decreased exercise capacity can be an early sign of magnesium deficiency. When the animals were given magnesium dissolved in water, their endurance was restored. Most human studies also confirm that both brief and extended exercise deplete magnesium.

THREE THINGS YOU NEED TO KNOW
ABOUT MAGNESIUM AND EXERCISE

1. Magnesium reduces lactic acid, which causes post-exercise pain.
2. Magnesium is lost during exercise.
3. Magnesium deficiency may cause sudden cardiac death in healthy athletes.

One of the most amazing effects of magnesium on the neuro-muscular system is that it provides more energy, even though the mineral generally acts as a relaxant and not a stimulant. If you are magnesium-deficient, your energy level will be low because you aren't producing the necessary energy to run your body. When you start taking magnesium, your energy level goes up. Magnesium's interactions with calcium help keep calcium from causing excessive muscle contraction. Excess calcium causes tension and tightness in all the muscles of the body, but when you take a balancing amount of magnesium, this tension releases within weeks, days, or even hours, depending on the underlying level of magnesium deficiency in your body.

Exercise is often prescribed therapeutically for anxiety and depression—to burn off steam (so to speak), to increase the circulation, and to get adrenaline pumping. Magnesium allows the body to burn fuel and create energy in an efficient cycle during exercise that does not lead to lactic acid production and buildup. For some individuals who exercise excessively or suffer from chronic fatigue syndrome, painful amounts of lactic acid build up in their muscles, making exercise an unpleasant experience. Exercise itself places stress on your body, to which your adrenal glands respond by pumping out adrenaline.

Heavy exercisers, especially long-distance runners, can build up lactic acid and suffer shin splints and painful muscles, but they keep on running because they may be addicted to the adrenaline rush they get when they reach "the wall" in their workout. The wall feels like something you just can't break through, but you keep on pushing, and suddenly you get a burst of adrenaline and you're flying. That's the power of your adrenal glands when pushed to the maximum. Yet that stress-induced high is followed by a crash when you don't repair the damage to your adrenal glands with good nutrition and restore the magnesium that was lost during exercise.

Many studies have shown that magnesium supplementation enhances the performance and endurance of long-distance runners, cross-country skiers, cyclists, and swimmers. It also reduces lactic acid buildup and postexercise cramps and pain. Since athletes undergo severe physical stress as well as the psychological drive to win, and most ingest suboptimal amounts of magnesium, they are vulnerable to magnesium deficiency.[17]

Years ago the coach of a Florida high school football team was concerned about his players' frequent complaints of leg cramps, so he gave them a calcium supplement on a very hot day before a rigorous game. Early in the second half, eleven players became disoriented and had difficulty walking. Their speech was slurred, they complained of muscle spasms, and they were breathing very deeply. Within an hour, eight of the boys collapsed into full-blown seizures; two had repeated seizures. Those having the worst symptoms had been playing the hardest. Thirteen more players reported headaches, blurred vision, muscle twitching, nausea, and weakness.[18] Eventually all the boys recovered, but what happened to create such a frightening scene in this group of healthy young men? Consider the facts. Those that were affected had all eaten a pregame magnesium-deficient fast-food meal consisting mainly of carbohydrates and fats, and sodas containing phosphoric acid. With the increased magnesium loss from excessive sweating plus the calcium supplement, their magnesium stores had been driven dangerously low.[19]

Magnesium deficiency may also play a role in sudden cardiac death syndrome, which can affect athletes.[20] In a study of young, healthy, well-conditioned men, strenuous effort was reported to give rise to persistent magnesium deficiency and a related long-term increase in cholesterol, triglycerides, and blood sugar. This study postulates that the sudden death of athletes and other intensely training individuals during extreme exertion is triggered by the detrimental effects of persistent magnesium deficiency on the cardiovascular system.[21, 22]

MAGNESIUM SUPPLEMENTS FOR EXERCISERS AND ATHLETES

Dr. Seelig, an internationally recognized magnesium specialist, recommends that athletes in training obtain at least 6–10 mg/kg/day (or 2.7–4.5 mg/lb/day) of magnesium to help replace the losses from exertion, sweating, and stress.

For a 220-lb man: 600–1,000 mg per day
For a 150-lb woman: 400–680 mg per day

These doses can be cut by 150 mg for people who exercise moderately (one to two hours a day).

—

CHAPTER FIVE

STROKES, HEAD INJURY, AND BRAIN SURGERY

THREE THINGS YOU NEED TO KNOW ABOUT MAGNESIUM AND THE BRAIN

---

1. Magnesium protects the brain from the toxic effects of chemicals such as food additives.
2. Magnesium keeps calcium out of cells; when magnesium is low, calcium rushes in, causing cell death.
3. When blood sugar and magnesium are both low, the glutamate in MSG enters brain cells, causing cell death.

Magnesium does much more than any drug to protect the blood circulation and the brain:

- It's a vasodilator, opening up blood vessels.
- It protects the endothelium, or inner layer of blood vessels.
- It closes the calcium channel to excessive calcium influx.

MAGNESIUM-DEFICIENT BRAINS

With most of the U.S. population deficient in magnesium,[1] many Americans are at greater risk for a host of serious problems, including stroke with severe poststroke complications, depending on the degree of magnesium deficiency; poor recovery from head injury with escalating neurological damage; neurotoxin damage from vast numbers of chemicals in our air, food, and water; seizure disorders; Alzheimer's disease; and Parkinson's disease.[2] These conditions are the neurological equivalent of heart disease. After all, both heart and brain are excitable tissues that give off electrical energy, and both must have magnesium. The complexity of the mechanisms of central nervous system hyperexcitability due to magnesium deficiency is only now being appreciated.[3]

HEAD INJURY AND MAGNESIUM

Traumatic brain injury (TBI) is a major public health problem throughout the world. There are more than 400,000 patients with TBI in the United States alone. From animal studies, we know that brain magnesium levels fall dramatically at the site of injury as this mineral is depleted in a cascade of events.[4] In sixty-six human subjects with acute blunt head trauma, the greater the degree of injury, the greater the calcium-ion-to-magnesium-ion ratio.

Such findings provide evidence of magnesium ion changes in the blood after traumatic brain injury, which could be of both diagnostic and prognostic value.[5] Studies of both animals and human brain trauma victims suggest that higher magnesium levels are associated with a better recovery.[6] Giving sufficient magnesium will create a better healing outcome. Magnesium sulfate significantly reduces brain edema following brain injury and is used to treat patients with severe TBI without adverse effects.[7] This is crucial information to give your doctor if your child suffers a head injury or any family member is involved in a motor vehicle accident.

Ionic magnesium testing, used in research studies, makes the diagnosis of posttraumatic headaches much easier. Abnormalities in magnesium ion concentration and the calcium-ion-to-magnesium-ion ratio were found in children with posttraumatic headaches, but serum magnesium levels were normal.[8] Obviously, studies using only the serum magnesium test would miss the diagnosis and fail to properly treat these patients. See Chapter 16 for a full discussion of magnesium testing.

A magnesium deficit from head injury is slow to reverse. According to neurosurgeon Dr. Russell Blaylock, magnesium takes thirty minutes to get into the spinal fluid, three hours to reach the cortical area directly under the skull, and a full four to six hours for sufficient amounts of magnesium to reach the deep brain tissues. Experiments with Navy SEALs and marathon runners show that after a month of intensive training, they experience magnesium deficiency and, if no supplements are taken, the deficiency is still present three to six months later. It only makes sense that if your diet is deficient and you're under stress, physical or emotional, you need to replace your magnesium stores daily.

BRAIN INJURY, ALCOHOL, AND MAGNESIUM

Drs. Bella and Burton Altura discuss the direct cause-and-effect relationship between alcohol-induced headache and risk of brain injury and stroke in one of their numerous papers.[9] They note that binge drinking of alcohol is associated with an ever-growing number of strokes and cases of sudden death,

with alcohol causing spasm and rupture of the cerebral arteries.[10] In animal studies, high doses of alcohol caused a rapid
fall in levels of magnesium ions in the brain and an elevation
of calcium, followed by cerebral vessel spasm and rupture of
cerebral blood vessels (stroke).[11, 12] People who consume more
than three alcoholic drinks a day can be deficient because alcohol blocks magnesium absorption.[13] In human studies, people with mild head injury have been found to exhibit early
deficits in magnesium ions; the greater the degree of head injury, the greater and more profound the deficit in magnesium
ions, and the greater the level of calcium ions compared to
magnesium ions. Patients with histories of alcohol abuse or ingestion of alcohol prior to head injury exhibited greater deficits
in magnesium ions (and higher calcium-ion-to-magnesium-
ion ratios) and, unlike the subjects without alcohol, remained
in the hospital at least several days longer. Data on 105 men
and women with different types of stroke indicate that, on average, a 20 percent deficit in magnesium ions is seen, while
serum magnesium is usually normal.[14]

As pointed out many times previously and also in Chapter 16, serum magnesium is a highly inaccurate measurement
of the body's magnesium because only 1 percent of the magnesium in the body resides in the blood. The Alturas also report that in other human studies, it has been shown that the
migraines, headache, dizziness, and hangover that accompany
alcohol ingestion are associated with rapid deficits in magnesium ion levels but not in serum magnesium, which obscures
the diagnosis if only serum magnesium is measured. And
since magnesium is necessary to regulate calcium, its deficiency creates calcium-induced vascular spasms and pathology.[15] Alcohol-associated headaches can be treated with
intravenous administration of magnesium sulfate.[16] Premenstrual tension headache and its exacerbation by alcohol in

women is also accompanied by deficits in magnesium ions and elevation in the calcium-ion-to-magnesium-ion ratio, and can be corrected by intravenous magnesium sulfate.

STROKE

A burst or clot-blocked blood vessel in the brain is all it takes to cause a stroke. The damage in so confined a space destroys critical brain functions. Stroke is said to be caused by hypertension, atherosclerosis, and diabetic complications—all of which are associated with low magnesium. Keeping blood vessels strong, preventing blood from clotting inappropriately, and even healing stroke-damaged areas are all within the scope of the miracle of magnesium.

Stroke has devastated the lives of 4.6 million Americans and 15 million people worldwide. Each year about 700,000 new strokes occur, along with 100,000 recurrences—and statisticians say that the incidence of stroke is on the rise.

What evidence is there of the importance of magnesium in stroke? All deaths due to stroke among Taiwan residents (17,133 cases) from 1989 through 1993 were compared with deaths from other causes (17,133 controls). It was determined that the higher the magnesium levels in drinking water used by the Taiwan residents, the lower the incidence of stroke.[17]

Animal experiments show that intravenous magnesium can prevent alcohol-induced hemorrhagic stroke and the subsequent fall in brain magnesium ion level as well as other metabolic factors.[18] Recent data indicate that alcohol-induced cellular loss of magnesium ions is associated with cellular calcium overload and generation of free radicals; however, pretreatment with vitamin E can also prevent alcohol-induced vascular injury and pathology in the brain.[19] (Learn more about free radicals on pages 199–201.)

What about humans? Can they benefit from IV magnesium for reversing symptoms of stroke? I interviewed Dan Haley, a former New York assemblyman, on this topic. Dan has spent over a decade researching alternative healing modalities and wrote a book called *Politics in Healing* (2000). When Dan suffered a stroke that paralyzed his entire left side in August 2004, one of his many connections advised him to immediately see a doctor in Washington, D.C., who offers IV magnesium and oxygen for this condition. Dan had already seen some improvement with several acupuncture treatments and could move his left hand, but his doctor had to go to China, so Dan went in the other direction, to Washington. Within ten days of receiving these daily treatments as an outpatient, Dan was walking and had full use of his left arm.[20]

Dr. Bruce Rind is Dan's Washington doctor. He and Dr. Sean Dalton developed the RELOX procedure for stroke, which consists of an intravenous vitamin mineral solution, with a heavy emphasis on magnesium, and the simultaneous application of oxygen by mask. In Dan's case, Dr. Rind added hour-long sessions in a hyperbaric oxygen chamber to further enhance the delivery of oxygen to the brain.

Drs. Dalton and Rind presented their RELOX protocol at the Neuroscience 2005 Conference in Washington, in November. The conference was attended by 30,000 people and honored with a keynote address by the Dalai Lama. In their talk, "Stroke Rehabilitation: An Investigation of Clinical and Neurological Recovery with a Nutrient-Oxygen Intervention," the doctors pointed out that there has been little research focused on the potential of cost-effective nutriceutical-biologic interventions to improve/restore clinical and neurological function in subacute-chronic stroke patients who are functioning with paralysis and no hope of cure. They told the audience that the RELOX procedure has been administered to a patient population of over 200 who have suffered the aftereffects of stroke from periods ranging from a few days to twenty-plus years.

Their results have been nothing less than miraculous. Patients with mild to moderate impairment experienced "moderate to significant, relatively sustained clinical recovery of cognitive, motor, and sensory functions after three 40-minute treatments with no significant adverse effects." SPECT scans of these patients suggested "cerebral functional volume recovery correlated with CBF (cerebral blood flow) and metabolic increases."

Contrary to most medical opinion, Drs. Rind and Dalton are proving that the area of stroke damage "may represent relatively viable, functionally depressed, albeit potentially salvageable regions for a more extended period following stroke or other cerebral insult than heretofore estimated."

The good doctors know this to be a real possibility because their procedure has helped the majority of patients treated. They remark, "Given the potentially remarkable personal, social, and economic benefits for patients and society, further investigation of the RELOX Procedure's clinical and neurological efficacy, safety, and mechanisms of action is warranted."

Drs. Rind and Dalton plan a pilot study of chronic stroke patients involving acute-subacute stroke, cerebral palsy, and traumatic brain injured patients. You can find their contact information in the Resources section.

BRAIN SURGERY AND MAGNESIUM

During and after brain surgery, magnesium's many attributes come into play by preventing stroke, keeping calcium from entering damaged cells, and decreasing the incidence of seizure and spasm. These favorable effects have all been proven unequivocally in animal studies, but clinical experience in the neurosurgical operating room also proves its efficacy as lives are being saved. Many surgeons make it standard procedure to administer intravenous magnesium to all their surgical patients before an operation. Dr. Bernard Horn, a general surgeon in California, has given intravenous magnesium sulfate to more than 8,000 patients over a fifteen-year period. Dr. Horn reports that blood pressures as high as 200 over 150 would normalize before surgery.[21]

Intravenous magnesium sulfate also acts as a general anesthetic so that during surgery the dose of other chemical anesthetics can be safely reduced. Using intravenous magnesium also results in lower postoperative pain scores, less pain medication needed in the twenty-four hours after surgery, and less postoperative nausea and vomiting. Magnesium sulfate is therefore a safe and cost-effective addition to such general anesthetics as propofol, remifentanil, and mivacurium.[22]

THREE THINGS YOU NEED TO KNOW ABOUT MAGNESIUM AND BRAIN SURGERY

1. Good neurosurgeons give magnesium to all their surgical patients.
2. Magnesium helps the brain recover from brain surgery.
3. Magnesium can prevent post-surgical strokes or make them less damaging.

Decades of research show that withdrawal of magnesium from cerebral arteries causes them to spasm, whereas elevated magnesium produces relaxation.[23, 24, 25] Animal studies show that when there is normal or elevated magnesium in the brain, the damage caused by stroke is reduced and the neurological deficit is lessened. This is because magnesium blocks calcium from flooding the cells and causing injury. Further research indicates that the area of the brain damaged by stroke contains injured neurons that remain hyperactive for several hours after the stroke has occurred.[26] These cells are frantically struggling to survive and need even more oxygen, glucose, and magnesium than normal. In addition, when these vital nutrients are deficient, those neurons become especially vulnerable to the damaging effects of excitotoxins that rush in to fill the void left by escaping nutrients. Hospitalized patients commonly have low magnesium levels, which means that neurons are even less likely to survive. According to one researcher, a state of severe magnesium deficiency alone is enough for rats to develop widespread injury to their brains, affecting key brain functions.[27]

A study of stroke patients in New York highlights the absolute requirement for magnesium intervention in the ER. Ninety-eight patients admitted to the emergency rooms of three hospitals with a diagnosis of stroke exhibited early and significant deficits in magnesium ions as measured with a sensitive ion-selective electrode. The stroke patients also demonstrated a high calcium-ion-to-magnesium-ion ratio, signs of increased vascular tone, and cerebral vessel spasm.[28]

MAGNESIUM AND SEIZURES

The brain is in a state of constant electrical activity. Brain cells are either stimulating or suppressing activity in a delicate push-and-pull balance. These cells are controlled by switches: some switches are turned on and some are turned off by neurotransmitters. The action of these neurotransmitters could not take place without calcium, magnesium, and zinc, which play various roles in the response of the nerve cells to electrical stimulation.

Brain cells altered by trauma, chemicals, or severe stress can be permanently switched on and fire excessively. Repeated firing in many nerve cells may result in seizures. Magnesium raises the threshold for seizures, reducing the chance of them developing at all. Conversely, experimental studies have shown that low magnesium in the body makes seizures more likely to occur.[29]

Magnesium sulfate for the treatment of seizures and hypertension in pregnancy is safe and effective and universally accepted. Unfortunately, large clinical trials using magnesium for other types of seizures and epilepsy has not been forthcoming. However, oral magnesium is used as an adjunct to antiepileptic medication by many practitioners.

≡

CHAPTER SIX

CHOLESTEROL AND HYPERTENSION

High cholesterol and hypertension are two conditions that plague Americans in epidemic proportions, and they appear to be the initial insults that lead to heart problems over time. But surprisingly, the real story behind both conditions could be a lack of magnesium.

CHOLESTEROL

There are several types of cholesterol with different functions; some of these types we label "good" and some "bad." High-density lipoprotein, HDL, is generally considered to be beneficial to the body; it helps remove cholesterol from blood vessel walls and the blood itself, bringing it to the liver for processing and excretion. Low-density lipoprotein, LDL, is harmful to the body because it carries cholesterol into the bloodstream, promoting the buildup of cholesterol plaque on the arterial walls. Very-low-density lipoproteins, VLDLs, are made into LDLs and therefore are harmful.

All of these cholesterols are normally found in the body. What's *not* normal is the high amounts of oxidized cholesterol

(cholesterol abnormally bound with oxygen) that we eat in processed foods, fast foods, and fried foods. In addition, chlorine, fluoride in water, pesticides, and other environmental pollutants can also oxidize cholesterol in the body. It is this oxidized cholesterol that researchers are concerned about when it comes to heart disease.[1]

Regular use of antioxidants such as magnesium, vitamin E, vitamin A, vitamin C, and green tea can lower oxidized cholesterol levels. There is compelling evidence that magnesium therapy reduces cholesterol levels,[2, 3, 4] even when there is a genetic risk factor present for hypercholesterolemia.[5]

Unfortunately, there are no visible physical symptoms of high cholesterol beyond the associated signs of a bad diet, sedentary lifestyle, smoking, alcohol intake, and stress. You have to find it on a blood test. A poor diet with a high intake of saturated and polyunsaturated fats, hydrogenated oils, fried foods, meat, sugar, coffee, and alcohol will elevate cholesterol levels, especially when a person lacks fiber from whole grains and vegetables. Add a sedentary lifestyle with weight gain, and cholesterol increases.

The very diet that promotes elevated cholesterol also causes magnesium deficiency. Unfortunately, many doctors do not have the time or inclination to educate patients about correct eating habits that could reduce their cholesterol; instead they rely on medication to treat the problem. To be fair, many patients don't have the inclination to comply even if their doctor recommends a change in diet, exercise, and weight loss. Adding magnesium supplementation to lifestyle changes, however, gives patients more dramatic improvement, making compliance easier.

Many of us have been conditioned to believe that elevated cholesterol is the only cause of heart disease; that is why marketers have been so successful in getting us to replace saturated fat such as butter with hydrogenated vegetable oils. Yet epidemiologists and dental anthropologists proved long ago that various world cultures that ate high-cholesterol diets for thousands of years (including meat, lard, cream, butter, and eggs) suffered very little, if any, heart disease.[6] Almost all the long-lived, healthy communities where degenerative disease and heart disease were unknown included significant amounts of natural, unprocessed meat or dairy in their diets. And it is also clear that once a country is exposed to refined and processed food, or "altered" meat and "altered" dairy, health declines in a number of ways.[7, 8, 9] Hydrogenated oils are unsaturated oils and for that reason were thought to be healthier than saturated fats such as butter. But the processing of liquid vegetable oil by heat, pressure, and chemicals to change it into a solid fat creates an unhealthy synthetic product called a trans fatty acid (as opposed to the natural cis fatty acid).

A major disadvantage of low-fat products is that they often contain extra sugar in order to capture the taste buds. Even worse is aspartame, a synthetic sweetener with a daunting list of side effects to its name. To maintain your health, avoid both.

Only in the late 1990s did research show that these highly refined hydrogenated oils themselves promote atherosclerotic plaque much more than butter. In fact, some scientists say that the rise of heart attacks, and heart disease in general, can be traced back to the late 1930s, when hydrogenated oils were first introduced. We now know that trans fatty acids cause arterial damage as well as cancer. Be sure to read labels to avoid this substance.

WHAT CHOLESTEROL DOES

Not just adults but every schoolchild has been conditioned to believe that cholesterol is the bad guy in heart disease. But did you know that without cholesterol we wouldn't be able to have sex, couldn't procreate, and would become extinct? That's simply because sex hormones and stress hormones are made from cholesterol. It's also necessary to create cell membranes and coat nerves with a protective fatty insulation that makes up about 60–80 percent of our brain tissue. Cholesterol is also essential for proper food digestion and fat absorption because it produces bile salts. Moreover, if you didn't have cholesterol, your bones would turn to mush because you couldn't make vitamin D from sunlight and wouldn't be able to absorb calcium.

If cholesterol is so crucial to life, why are we trying so desperately to get rid of it? In fact, our body thinks cholesterol is so important that the liver makes about 1,000 mg of cholesterol a day; if we try to lower our cholesterol too much with drugs, the liver merely gears up production. Normally, the liver produces about 85 percent of the cholesterol measured on a blood test. The other 15 percent comes from our diet.

WHEN CHOLESTEROL BECAME THE BAD GUY

In 1913, two Russian researchers fed large amounts of cholesterol to a group of hungry rabbits. When they saw yellow gunk clogging the rabbits' arteries, they leapt to the conclusion that cholesterol must be responsible for coronary artery disease.[10]

Robert Ford, as long ago as 1969, called the cholesterol theory of heart disease a tragic blunder.[11] In a book called *Stale Food vs. Fresh Food*, he gave us some important information about the Russian experiment that had been overlooked. He wrote, "Their finding was one of those unfortunate half-truths which only served to mislead." In his commonsense way of looking at the cholesterol theory of heart disease, Ford said, "It is absurd to say that something we are largely made of would be harmful for us to eat."

Ford explained that dietary cholesterol is harmful only if it is stale or rancid. When he read the original article by the Russians he was amazed to discover that they had fed their rabbits "pure crystalline cholesterol dissolved in vegetable oil" to produce the cholesterol buildup in arteries. They didn't stop to think that crystalline cholesterol is not something the body can use but is "an unnatural stale substance now known as oxycholesterol, which is not found in fresh food or in the healthy human body." Ford said the cholesterol theory is untrue and has served to deceive us by delaying discovery of the true causes and cures.

Udo Erasmus wrote an enlightening book about fats and oils called *Fats That Heal, Fats That Kill.* From his decades-long research he concludes, "The cholesterol scare is big business for doctors, laboratories, and drug companies. It is also a powerful marketing gimmick for vegetable oil and margarine manufacturers. In the end, cholesterol will be exonerated from its role as primary villain in cardiovascular disease. The accusing finger points at 'experts' who concocted the cholesterol theory to drum up business by spreading fear."[12]

THE DRUG TREATMENT OF CHOLESTEROL

Statins are a group of powerful drugs that block a specific enzyme in the liver that helps make cholesterol. When that enzyme is blocked, cholesterol levels are lowered. That enzyme, however, does much more in the body than just make cholesterol, so when it is suppressed by statins there are far-ranging consequences.

One major side effect that medicine acknowledges is elevated liver enzymes. Because statins work on liver enzymes, they can disrupt liver function. If you take statins, you must have regular blood tests to look for liver damage; stopping statins if your liver is damaged usually reverses the problem.

Another acknowledged side effect, statin myopathy, is an iatrogenic (doctor-induced) condition that damages muscles and is entirely related to statin intake. Statins cause a kind of muscle cell destruction called rhabdomyolysis, leading to muscle pain and tenderness. Myoglobin is a muscle protein that is released into the bloodstream and can be measured as a sign of statin myopathy. Interestingly, about 40 percent of the magnesium in the body is found in muscles, and magnesium is the mineral component of myosin (a large protein that forms skeletal muscle). So when muscle is destroyed, magnesium is lost from its storage site.

An unacknowledged side effect of statins is that they inhibit the production of coenzyme Q_{10}, which is a fat-soluble antioxidant found in large amounts in mitochondria. Mitochondria are the principle powerhouse of cells, where all the energy in the body is produced. You've already read about magnesium being necessary for the formation of ATP; it is in the mitochondria where this activity occurs. When the activity of mitochondria is damaged, as it is by statins, more than the energy of the body is diminished. Lowered levels of coenzyme Q_{10} may be the cause of the muscle damage called myopathy and also produces neuropathy (damage to nerves), memory decline including global amnesia, and cardiomyopathy (destruction of heart muscle).

Treatment of statin side effects includes high doses of coenzyme Q_{10}, 100 mg twice daily. However, what might work even better is to use magnesium as your first line of treatment for elevated cholesterol so you don't have to touch statin drugs at all.

MAGNESIUM ACTS LIKE A NATURAL STATIN

A well-known magnesium proponent, Mildred Seeling, M.D., just before she died in 2004, wrote a fascinating paper with Andrea Rosanoff, Ph.D., showing that magnesium acts by the same mechanisms as statin drugs to lower cholesterol.[13]

Every metabolic activity in the body depends on enzymes. Making cholesterol, for example, requires a specific enzyme called HMG-CoA reductase. As it turns out, magnesium slows down this enzymatic reaction when it is present in sufficient quantities. HMG-CoA reductase is the same enzyme that statin drugs target and inhibit. The mechanisms are nearly the same; however, magnesium is the natural way that the body has evolved to control cholesterol when it reaches a certain level, whereas statin drugs are used to destroy the whole process. This means that if sufficient magnesium is present in the body, cholesterol will be limited to its necessary functions—the production of hormones and the maintenance of membranes—and will not be produced in excess.

It's only in our present-day circumstances of magnesium-deficient soil, little magnesium in processed foods, and excessive intake of calcium and calcium-rich foods without supplementation of magnesium that cholesterol has become elevated in the population. If there is not enough magnesium to limit the activity of the cholesterol-converting enzyme, we are bound to make more cholesterol than is needed.

The magnesium/cholesterol story gets even better. Magnesium is responsible for several other lipid-altering functions that are not even shared by statin drugs. Magnesium is necessary for the activity of an enzyme that lowers LDL, the "bad" cholesterol; it also lowers triglycerides and raises the "good" cholesterol, HDL. Another magnesium-dependent enzyme converts omega-3 and omega-6 essential fatty acids into prostaglandins, which are necessary for heart and overall health.

Seelig and Rosanoff conclude their paper by saying that it is well accepted that magnesium is a natural calcium channel blocker, and now we know it also acts like a natural statin. In their book *The Magnesium Factor,* Seelig and Rosanoff reported that eighteen human studies verified that magnesium supplements can have an extremely beneficial effect on lipids. In these studies, total cholesterol levels were reduced by 6 to 23 percent; LDL (bad) cholesterol were lowered by 10 to 18 percent; tryglycerides fell by 10 to 42 percent; and HDL (good) cholesterol rose by 4 to 11 percent. Furthermore, the studies showed that low magnesium levels are associated with higher levels of "bad" cholesterol and and high magnesium levels indicate an increase in "good" cholesterol.

NORMAL LIPID VALUES

Cholesterol: 180–220 mg/dl
HDL cholesterol: greater than 45 mg/dl
LDL cholesterol: less than 130 mg/dl
VLDL cholesterol: less than 35 mg/dl
Total-cholesterol-to-HDL ratio: in men the optimal ratio is less than 3.43 (average 4.97); in women the optimal ratio is less than 3.27 (average 4.44)

THE LINK BETWEEN OXIDIZED CHOLESTEROL AND HOMOCYSTEINE

When Russian researchers showed that oxidized cholesterol causes blocked arteries, instead of learning from that message that oxidized cholesterol might be the problem, everyone assumed all cholesterol was bad. One process that produces oxidized cholesterol in the body is described by Dr. Kilmer McCully.

He was the first researcher, back in 1969, to identify a condition of increased levels of an amino acid, homocysteine, in the urine of patients with heart disease, which could be reversed with certain nutrients.[14, 15]

Homocysteine is a normal by-product of protein digestion, which in elevated amounts causes the oxidization of cholesterol—and it is oxidized cholesterol that damages blood vessels. For certain individuals who lack specific enzymes for protein digestion, homocysteine can become a real problem.

A healthy level of homocysteine is below 12 µmol/L. Homocysteine levels greater than 12 µmol/L are considered high, and when homocysteine is elevated in the cell, magnesium measures low. Twenty to 40 percent of the general population have elevated levels of homocysteine. Individuals with high levels have almost four times the risk of suffering a heart attack compared to people with normal levels.[16] Elevated homocysteine is high on the list of risk factors for heart disease and serves as an even stronger marker than high cholesterol for heart disease and blood clotting disorders.[17, 18]

The more relevant marker may be low magnesium since the major enzymes involved in homocysteine metabolism are magnesium-dependent.[19] McCully blames too much protein in the diet for elevated homocysteine. However, when magnesium, vitamin B_6, vitamin B_{12}, and folic acid are deficient, the body is not able to properly digest protein. The B vitamins were readily available in the typical diet a hundred years ago; now that they're absent from the diet, homocysteine becomes elevated and heart disease results.

When these metabolic nutrients are reintroduced through diet or supplements, the high homocysteine levels are reversed and the symptoms of heart disease diminish. Ongoing research confirms that B_6, B_{12}, and folic acid together with magnesium are necessary to prevent blood vessel damage induced by high levels of homocysteine in the blood.[20] In short, the successful treatment of homocysteinuria relies on dietary changes that include B vitamins and magnesium.[21, 22, 23] However, magnesium is often left out of the prescription for homocysteinuria in favor of the B vitamins—a common but serious error on the part of conventional medicine.

It must be remembered that high homocysteine is also a marker for all causes of mortality, which underscores that a deficiency in essential nutrients has a far-reaching effect on the body far beyond heart disease.[24]

HYPERTENSION

Hypertension is an elevation of blood pressure suffered by more than 50 million Americans. Most often, hypertension is diagnosed during a routine physical exam. It presents no distinguishing signs or symptoms unless the condition is very advanced, in which case headache, dizziness, and blurred vision can occur.

Normal blood pressure is a range: 100–140 over 60–90. Systolic pressure is the first number and relates to the pump pressure that the heart muscle creates to push blood into the arteries. Diastolic pressure is the second number and is the pressure that the arteries maintain when the heart is relaxed, between heartbeats, to keep the arteries open.

Hypertension is either primary or secondary. Primary hypertension is said to have no single cause and occurs in 90 percent of all hypertensive patients. Secondary hypertension is secondary to another disease. Causes of primary hypertension include high cholesterol, family history, obesity, diet, smoking, stress, and excessive salt intake—but one major cause that is overlooked is magnesium deficiency.

The necessity to keep blood pressure as low as possible may be another myth of modern medicine, just like cholesterol. In the past decade the value for high blood pressure has been lowered to the point that a majority of Americans fall in what's now called a prehypertensive category. When people are told they are prehypertensive, they don't hear the "pre-" part they just hear "hypertensive," and it scares them—sometimes enough to elevate their blood pressure, much like in what's called white-coat syndrome. This syndrome has your heart beating faster and your blood pressure rising because you are afraid your doctor will tell you that your blood pressure is elevated. Normal at home but high in the doctor's office is white-coat syndrome, not hypertension.

Certainly, high blood pressure is to be avoided, but these new values for normal blood pressure make it appear that almost everyone is susceptible to high blood pressure and should be on drugs. With the elderly and their slightly rigid blood vessels, a somewhat elevated blood pressure may be necessary to keep blood pumping to their head and extremities—and attempting to achieve a lower blood pressure in such individuals may perhaps cause dizziness and falls that could otherwise be prevented. A much more expedient solution is weight loss, exercise, stress reduction, and magnesium to prevent hypertension.

DRUGS FOR BLOOD PRESSURE

Diuretics are the first drugs on the recipe list for high blood pressure. These drugs help flush water from the body according to the theory that if there is less salt and water in your bloodstream, then there is less pressure on your blood vessels. But how is a doctor supposed to know if a patient has too much water in the bloodstream without doing complicated tests? And if you get rid of too much water, doesn't that make you dehydrated, thicken your blood, and make you susceptible to clotting-related conditions such as strokes and deep-vein thromboses?

Dr. Batmanghelidj, in his book *Your Body's Many Cries*

for Water, says that dehydration *causes* high blood pressure.[25] When the body is even slightly dehydrated, it attempts to hold on to whatever water it can by constricting blood vessels throughout the body. You sweat less and lose less moisture when you breathe—but constricted blood vessels mean increased blood pressure.

Dehydration is very common; most people don't drink enough water anyway, so why squeeze out more with a diuretic? When patients are prescribed diuretics, they are warned that the most common side effect is a deficiency of potassium, which spills out in the urine. To prevent it, they are advised to eat bananas and oranges or take potassium pills. What they are not told is that magnesium is drained out along with potassium. Recall that magnesium deficiency leads to blood vessels that are less relaxed and more susceptible to spasm and tension, a precursor to hypertension; thus the very treatment for hypertension worsens the problem.[26] (Ironically, replacing potassium doesn't help patients who are also magnesium-deficient, because the body is unable to deliver potassium to the cells without sufficient magnesium. Even the so-called potassium-sparing diuretics still commonly deplete other minerals, including magnesium.)[27] The common side effects of diuretics include weakness, muscle cramps, joint pain, and irregular heartbeat. They are also symptoms of magnesium deficiency. Proper testing for red blood cell magnesium should be a routine procedure when you are taking diuretics, but it currently is not.

DIURETICS DRY OUT THE BRAIN

A journal case study reported that an elderly woman's serum magnesium level became depleted due to a diuretic she was taking for hypertension.[28] She was admitted to the hospital with severe weakness and developed an overt psychosis with paranoid delusions. Fortunately, her magnesium deficiency was identified, and following large intravenous doses of magnesium, her symptoms disappeared within twenty-four hours. However, she was unable to discontinue magnesium therapy without a recurrence of her symptoms as long as she was taking the diuretic. No other abnormalities were found to explain her condition. People who are prescribed diuretics should check with their doctor about taking at least 600 mg a day of supplemental magnesium in divided doses. In that way, many of the side effects of diuretics can be avoided.

THE BLOOD PRESSURE RECIPE

If blood pressure is not controlled with diuretics, the next choice may be ACE inhibitors, calcium channel blockers, antiadrenergic drugs, or vasodilators. The treatment of high blood pressure by an internist friend provides a good example of "recipe medicine." I arrived early for an interview with my doctor friend and he invited me to sit in on an appointment with a very stressed, overweight newspaper reporter who was suffering from intractable high blood pressure in spite of being on a total of four different blood pressure medications. The patient said he was becoming depressed and was very concerned about his blood pressure. I recognized that the medications he was on could cause depression, as could the stress of having a case of high blood pressure that does not respond to treatment. But I also asked about impotence, suspecting this side effect of his drugs as a possible cause of his depression. He said he had been suffering impotence since going on the medications but had attributed it to stress.

As I noted earlier, the patient was overweight. When I asked about diet, the doctor admitted that he hadn't offered specific diet advice to the patient but did tell him to try to lose weight. I also mentioned the usefulness of magnesium as a mineral that excels as a natural antihypertensive, muscle relaxant, antianxiety remedy, and sleep aid. The doctor said that if the four different types of antihypertensive drugs don't help a patient, he will add magnesium, and it always works. Only professional courtesy kept me from shouting, "Why not prescribe the magnesium first, before all the other drugs with their nasty side effects?"

Fortunately, a growing number of internists and cardiologists know that magnesium is a physiological necessity and a pharmacological treasure to use before drug intervention. They call magnesium the ideal drug: it is safe, cheap, and simple to use, with a wide therapeutic range, a short half-life, and little or no tendency toward drug interactions.[29]

WEIGHT LOSS DROPS BLOOD PRESSURE

Long before drugs are introduced, diet should be the first treatment of choice for hypertension. Research shows a direct relationship between the amount of magnesium in the diet and the ability to avoid high blood pressure.[30] The Alturas first demonstrated that diets deficient in magnesium will produce hypertension in experimental animals.[31] Diet may lower the blood pressure successfully due to a combination of weight loss and increased intake of the vitamin and mineral cofactors necessary in blood pressure control. For example, increased levels of minerals such as potassium and magnesium in the diet have a suppressive effect on calcium-regulating hormones, which influence blood pressure.[32] The arterial blood pressure appears to go up as the levels of magnesium ions and serum magnesium go down.[33]

Weight loss is given only a passing mention in most clinical textbooks on blood pressure. The authors in these texts admit that if you can get a person to lose weight, then his or her blood pressure will usually go down. Every study that's been done on this subject reports this association. However, most doctors say that because they have little success with helping their patients lose weight, they often offer medications as the first line of treatment. Doctors have two strikes against them when it comes to weight loss: they receive no training in weight loss management in medical school, and health insurance does not pay for nutritional counseling or prevention of disease—it pays only when there is a disease code.

Note: Some forms of severe high blood pressure are hereditary or due to kidney disease and do require medication. Also, if the arteries in the body are damaged from long-term atherosclerotic injury and scarring, unfortunately they may no longer respond to magnesium and you may require medications to keep your blood pressure under control.

For information on magnesium supplements for hypertension, see "Supplements for Heart Disease" on pages 115–116.

CHAPTER SEVEN

MAGNESIUM AND HEART DISEASE

THREE THINGS YOU NEED TO KNOW
ABOUT MAGNESIUM AND HEART DISEASE

1. Magnesium prevents muscle spasms of the heart blood vessels, which can lead to heart attack.
2. Magnesium prevents muscle spasms of the peripheral blood vessels, which can lead to high blood pressure.
3. Magnesium prevents calcium buildup in cholesterol plaque in arteries, which leads to clogged arteries.

Annette was tired of people's shocked reaction when they learned that she was recovering from a heart attack. She knew that the common image of heart disease was that it afflicted aggressive, overweight men who smoked and ate too much. Annette, on the other hand, was slim, reserved, and a vegetarian who ate a low-fat diet. She chuckled when friends tried to tell her about the Dr. Dean Ornish vegetarian diet for reversing heart disease, because she'd lived according to that diet.

She was only fifty-six, a nonsmoker, with exemplary cholesterol levels, but she did have elevated blood pressure, her only risk factor. And, as she was told by her doctor, because of her blood pressure, she had had a mild heart attack. Now she suffered from daily palpitations and was on several medications that seemed to drain her energy more with every passing day. She was also simply too afraid to exert herself for fear of bringing on another heart attack.

Annette was becoming an invalid, and at her next appointment her cardiologist was shocked at her worn-out appearance. He decided to run some blood tests and was urged by a student doctor to order a red blood cell magnesium test. The results of that test were so low that his nurse immediately called Annette to come in, saying the doctor had found something that would help her feel better. Annette was prescribed a magnesium preparation that she mixed with water (Slow-Mag) that began to work within twenty-four hours. She was amazed that her muscle aches, insomnia, palpitations, and fatigue all but disappeared. She was even able to cut back on her other medications. Her doctor vowed to test all his patients' magnesium red blood cell levels from then on, and wondered aloud if it had been low magnesium in the first place that had led to Annette's heart attack.

AN IMPORTANT REMINDER ABOUT TAKING
MAGNESIUM WITH PRESCRIPTION DRUGS

You may experience a decreased need for your drugs as magnesium deficiency is corrected or as magnesium treats your symptoms or reverses your condition. In other words, the symptoms for which the drug was prescribed may clear up due to the magnesium, making the drug unnecessary or toxic and causing new symptoms. Patients and doctors should be on the alert for a shift in symptoms. Be sure to work with your doctor to lower your medication doses safely.

A 2003 study gives doctors all the evidence they need to include magnesium in their protocol for women suffering heart disease. The findings from this study show that "dietary magnesium depletion can be induced in otherwise healthy women; it results in increased energy needs and adversely affects cardiovascular function during submaximal work."[1]

As we will learn in Chapter 10, obstetricians are quite familiar with the use of magnesium for hypertension in women about to deliver. Unfortunately, they aren't talking to cardiologists or even to family doctors about the importance of magnesium in treating general hypertension, one of the main risk factors for heart disease, or using magnesium to prevent heart problems.

Heart disease is the number one killer of both American women and men, accounting for half of all U.S. deaths (52.3 percent of the total deaths occurring in women, compared to 47.7 percent in men). According to the American Heart Association, every thirty-three seconds someone in the United States dies of cardiovascular disease; that's approaching 1 million deaths annually. Hypertension occurs in 50 million Americans and accounts for an estimated 29.3 million office visits a year to conventional medical doctors.[2] Prescriptions for antihypertensive drugs are given at most of these appointments, even though magnesium has been used successfully for over half a century by medical doctors, osteopaths, and naturopathic doctors.[3, 4]

THE SLIPPERY ROAD TO HEART ATTACK

STEP ONE: LOSS OF ARTERIAL ELASTICITY
The coronary arteries bringing oxygen-filled blood from inside the heart through the aorta to the heart muscle are very,

very small, only about 3 mm across (a nickel is 2 mm thick). It doesn't take much to plug them up with a tiny blood clot or to cause them to collapse when in spasm. Magnesium prevents blood clot formation and artery spasm. These blood vessels get even smaller as they split into two, then four, then eight, and so on as they descend toward the bottom of the heart; some of the tiniest capillaries are only the width of a red blood cell. Each of these splits is called a bifurcation. According to cardiologists, about 85 percent of sclerotic plaques initially form near bifurcations. It is widely believed that the development of these plaques is a response to injury. This means that something, such as an infection, may be damaging the arteries, initiating the buildup of fat and calcium around the inflammation.

Endothelial cells are a single layer of specialized cells that form the inside membrane of an artery. The subendothelial layer (the next layer in) is a very thin connective tissue that contains elastin. As its name implies, this is the layer responsible for providing much of the elasticity in your arteries. It is important to note that your body requires magnesium to maintain healthy elastin. One of the earliest signs of magnesium deficiency is degeneration of elastin in the subendothelium.

Smooth muscle cells are the next layer. Smooth muscle cells provide integrity and control the dilation of the arterial cavity, triggered by the calcium/magnesium ratio in the body. Calcium causes contraction and magnesium causes relaxation, which together control the blood pressure and flow in the artery. A final messenger for the dilation response is nitric oxide, which is dependent on magnesium. Animals on low-magnesium diets lose the elasticity of their arterial system. Coronary arteries require even more elasticity than other arteries because they must stretch and flex as the heart expands and contracts. Loss of elasticity results in inflammation of the endothelial and subendothelial layers at the points that are most mechanically challenged by stretching: the bifurcations. Imagine a small rubber-band-like tube shaped like a Y. In your mind's eye grasp the two legs of the Y in one hand. With your other hand, grip the single leg. Begin pulling them apart just as though they were stretching on the surface of the heart. Stretch it as far as you can. Where is the shape weakest? If we left the rubber tube out in the sun for a week or so, what would happen if you slowly stretched it again? Where might you expect the first crack to appear? Most of the time it would happen at or near where one tube becomes two—at the bifurcation. If your artery loses elasticity, it makes sense that the problem might show up at or near the bifurcation.

STEP TWO: THE INFLAMMATORY RESPONSE

Inflammation begins with injury of the artery wall, leading to white blood cells and cholesterol hovering around trying to heal the damage. At this stage in the process, if there is too much calcium and not enough magnesium in the bloodstream, excess calcium precipitates around the area of inflammation in the artery wall. The area becomes rigid and interferes with blood flow.

STEP THREE: HEART ATTACK

Over time, the above steps weaken and plug the coronary arteries and slowly destroy small areas of the heart muscle. The final result is severe chest pain, damage to a larger portion of heart muscle, and heart attack.[5]

Some of the first evidence for the use of magnesium against heart disease came from epidemiological studies in Wales, Taiwan, Sweden, Finland, and Japan showing that death rates from coronary heart disease are higher in communities with magnesium-deficient water and magnesium-deficient diets.[6] Areas where calcium in the water is much higher than magnesium or where dietary intake of calcium is higher than magnesium showed even more coronary heart disease. A U.S. study done over a seven-year period followed 14,000 men and women and concluded that low magnesium in the diet may contribute to coronary atherosclerosis and acute heart attack.[7]

The Centers for Disease Control and Prevention in Atlanta followed 12,000 people for nineteen years, at the end of which 4,282 people had died, 1,005 from heart disease. Risk of dying from heart disease was highest in those with magnesium deficiency. Researchers made a conservative estimate that 11 percent of the half million deaths related to heart disease in 1993 could have been directly related to magnesium deficiency.[8] If more accurate measurements for magnesium deficiency were used, such as ionic magnesium testing, we would find the numbers to be even higher and the need for magnesium even greater.

The evidence has been mounting for decades that magnesium plays a crucial role in the prevention of both atherosclerosis and arteriosclerosis.[9, 10] It maintains the elasticity of the artery wall, dilates blood vessels, prevents calcium deposits, and is necessary for the maintenance of healthy muscles, including the heart muscle itself. For all these reasons, magnesium is critical to the maintenance of a healthy heart.[11] One of the pivotal metabolic chemicals in the body is nitric oxide (NO). It is a very simple compound made from nitrogen and oxygen, but it packs a powerful punch. Nitric oxide controls vasodilation, but this activity is under the direction of magnesium.[12]

C-REACTIVE PROTEIN

A December 2005 study confirms that C-reactive protein (CRP) has emerged as one of the most powerful predictors of heart disease.[13] In time, as more research is done, CRP will probably supplant cholesterol as the most significant predictor. Why is this important? Because CRP is an indicator of inflammation—and as previously noted, it's the injury and inflammation of heart blood vessels that underlie heart disease. The 2005 study also examines uric acid and finds that this product of protein breakdown, which is associated with hypertension, inflammation, and heart disease, also damages blood vessel walls. This action is mediated by nitric oxide and causes elevated CRP. These findings heighten the important role of magnesium in the process. Sufficient magnesium can hinder the pathology at every stage, whereas anti-inflammatory prescription drugs are ineffective and can carry dangerous side effects. An optimal level of CRP is less than 6 mg/l.

A U.S. study, reported in the July 2006 issue of the journal *Nutrition Research*, found that a daily magnesium supplement could reduce the levels of inflammation, as measured by C-reactive protein, that could lead to heart disease in people with low dietary intake of the mineral. This is very encouraging news in the fight against the single largest killer in the United States. It's also encouraging that researchers are investigating magnesium supplementation and not just dietary magnesium. In this study of over 10,000 people, only 21 percent were getting the RDA for magnesium in their diet. Another 26 percent were taking magnesium supplements, and it was that group that exhibited a lower C-reactive protein than the magnesium-deficient group.

ATHEROSCLEROSIS

It is easy to confuse the terms *arteriosclerosis* and *atherosclerosis:* in fact, many people use them interchangeably. *Arteriosclerosis* is the overall term for scarring of the arteries. *Atherosclerosis* is scarring or thickening specifically due to fatty plaques. When the diameter of an artery is already narrowed by fat deposits, a blood clot or an arterial spasm can be the final straw that results in angina, heart attack, or stroke. Complications of this preventable condition of atherosclerosis cause over a third of all deaths in the United States.

SUPPLEMENT AND DRUG INTERACTIONS
IN HEART DISEASE

1. Calcium interacts with verapamil (Calan, Isoptin, Vere-lan). Verapamil is a calcium channel blocker, and calcium interferes with the hypotensive effect of this drug. Avoid calcium until your doctor weans you off this drug.

2. Vitamin B_1 (thiamine) interacts with furosemide (Lasix). Lasix causes increased urinary excretion of B_1, so supplements of this vitamin may be necessary.

3. Vitamin B_6 interacts with hydralazine (Alazine, Apresazide, Apresoline, Unipres). Hydralazine causes increased excretion of vitamin B_6; supplements of the nutrient may be necessary.

4. Calcium, magnesium, and potassium interact with furosemide (Lasix), which causes urinary excretion of these minerals. Monitor levels of these nutrients and replace as necessary.

5. Grapefruit juice makes felodipine (Plendil) and nifedipine (Adalat, Procardia) more powerful; it increases the action of these drugs by temporarily blocking the enzyme that clears them from the body. You may have to avoid grapefruit juice while on these medications.

6. Magnesium, calcium, potassium, and sodium interact with thiazide diuretics such as chlorothiazide (Diuril, Diachlor) and hydrochlorothiazide (Aldoril, Hydrodiuril).

    Thiazides work by increasing urinary excretion of sodium, which presumably lowers blood pressure. However, significant amounts of calcium, potassium, and magnesium are also excreted. Magnesium at 600 mg per day may have to be increased to 900 mg if you are on thiazide diuretics or digitalis because both drugs cause excretion of magnesium. Your doctor should do a red blood cell magnesium test or EXATest to determine your needs. (See Chapter 16 for more on magnesium testing.)

7. Potassium and magnesium deficiencies lead to arrhythmias in patients on digoxin (Lanoxin).

8. Small increases in plasma calcium increase digoxin (Lanoxin) toxicity. Some specialists advise avoiding high-calcium foods for two hours before and after taking this drug.

9. Calcium should be supplemented due to decreased absorption of vitamin D with patients using the cholesterol-lowering drugs colestipol (Colestid) or cholestyramine (Questran).

10. Colestipol (Colestid) interferes with absorption of iron, folate, and vitamins A, D, E, and K.

11. Cholestyramine (Questran) interferes with absorption of iron, folate, and vitamins A, D, E, and K.

12. Heparin interferes with renal hydroxylation of vitamin D. This could lead to osteopenia; your doctor may need to check your vitamin D status with a 25-hydroxy vitamin D test, also called 25(O++)D.

13. Vitamin K inactivates warfarin (Coumadin); warfarin interferes with vitamin K synthesis.[14]

Researchers have identified various causes of damage to the inner wall of arteries, including homocysteine, an amino acid discussed earlier that creates oxidized cholesterol; infection by an organism called chlamydia; distorted blood flow around the mound of fat; free radicals; high blood sugar; high blood pressure; and lack of oxygen. As described previously, the damaged tissue of the artery wall initiates an inflammatory process. The inflammation then attracts "bad" cholesterol (LDL) and calcium, which build up into a solid scar. Magnesium has a role to play in reducing homocysteine levels, preventing free radicals, balancing blood sugar, and reducing high blood pressure.

ANGINA

Angina describes an episodic pain in the region of the chest and/or down the left arm due to lack of oxygen to the heart muscle and a buildup of carbon dioxide and other metabolites. Usually the pain, which can be a mild ache, pressure, or fullness, or a crushing pain, comes on with exercise (especially in the cold), emotional stress, a heavy meal, or even a vivid dream, and is relieved (usually within five minutes) by rest and nitroglycerine.

The lack of sufficient blood flow carrying life-giving oxygen and nutrients can be due to blocked coronary arteries or spasms in these tiny vessels. Angina is labeled "unstable" when symptoms become more severe; unstable angina implies a greater risk for heart attack. Another type of angina is called Prinzmetal's, which is angina that occurs at rest, rather than following some sort of physical stress. James B. Pierce, Ph.D., believes he has identified the cause of Prinzmetal's, which occurs most commonly at two specific times in the day, early morning and late afternoon, coincidentally when magnesium levels are at their lowest.[15] Dr. Pierce estimates that up to 50 percent of sudden heart attacks may be due to magnesium deficiency. He found that magnesium worked better than nitroglycerine for his own stress-induced chest pains. In fact, Dr. Pierce could predict that he would get chest pain after a stressful day, a long drive, or an emotional upset and would increase his intake of magnesium to forestall symptoms.

Risk factors for angina include magnesium deficiency, smoking, diabetes mellitus, hyperlipidemia, type A personality, sedentary lifestyle, poor diet, and family history of coronary artery disease. Diagnosis of angina, to differentiate it from myocardial infarction and unstable angina, includes an EKG (electrocardiogram) taken during an angina attack; an exercise tolerance test, which is an EKG taken while on a treadmill; and a coronary angiogram (an X-ray view of dye in the coronary arteries) to assess whether the coronary arteries are open or blocked.

Once angina is diagnosed, the recommendations are universally known: stop smoking, lose weight, get blood pressure under control (with or without drugs), and in extreme cases of arterial blockages, undergo bypass surgery to circumvent blocked arteries. The best treatment for angina, however, is prevention. By eliminating sugar, alcohol, and junk food from your diet you help prevent heart disease, because these foods are lacking in magnesium and serve only to create magnesium deficiency. When you eat a more balanced, non-processed-food diet, you have a better chance of increasing your magnesium intake. With magnesium and other heart-healthy supplements, a healthy diet, and an exercise regimen, you have a fighting chance of avoiding this epidemic. See pages 115–16 for a list of supplements to cover all aspects of heart disease.

HEART ATTACKS

Myocardial infarction (MI), or heart attack, causes permanent damage to the heart muscle and requires immediate hospitalization. MI is the result of coronary artery disease due to atherosclerosis or due to spasms caused or aggravated by magnesium deficiency. The artery may be damaged gradually by plaque, become blocked by a blood clot, or both, and suddenly go into spasm; either of these processes can be accelerated by excessive emotion. The calcified atherosclerotic plaque, the blood clot, and the arterial spasm all can be caused or worsened by magnesium deficiency.

Laboratory findings distinguish a heart attack from an

episode of angina on the basis of heart muscle damage and certain heart enzyme levels that become elevated several hours after a heart attack and remain elevated for several days. The immediate treatment for an acute heart attack usually includes anticoagulant drugs in an intravenous drip. Intravenous magnesium given as soon as possible after a heart attack, however, may provide the best protection for the heart. Oral magnesium treatment also inhibits blood clots in patients with coronary artery disease whether the patient is on aspirin therapy or not.[16] As more doctors read the considerable research on magnesium they are incorporating magnesium into their intravenous and oral protocols for heart patients.

Magnesium has been studied for its effects on the heart since the 1930s and used by injection for the treatment of heart conditions since the 1940s.[17, 18] Magnesium's lifesaving effects have been confirmed and reconfirmed in many clinics and laboratories. For example, in an analysis of seven major clinical studies, researchers concluded that magnesium (in doses of 5–10 g by intravenous injection) reduced the odds of death by an astounding 55 percent in acute MI.[19, 20] Over the past decade, several large clinical trials using magnesium have shown its beneficial effects: if intravenous magnesium is given (1) before any other drugs and (2) immediately after onset of a heart attack, the incidence of high blood pressure, congestive heart failure, arrhythmia, or a subsequent heart attack is vastly reduced. One such study, called LIMIT-2, provided powerful evidence that early magnesium administration protects the heart muscle, prevents arrhythmia, and improves long-term survival.[21, 22, 23] Magnesium might improve the aftermath of acute heart attack by preventing rhythm problems; improving blood flow to the heart by dilating blood vessels; protecting the damaged heart muscle against calcium overload; improving heart muscle function; breaking down any blood clots blocking the arteries; and reducing free radical damage. Magnesium may also help the heart drug digoxin to be more effective in the treatment of cardiac arrhythmia;[24] without enough magnesium, digoxin can become toxic.[25]

The suggested criteria for magnesium intervention were not followed in a very large trial called ISIS-4, and the outcome did not show the same results as the LIMIT trial.[26] In the ISIS trial, magnesium was given many hours after the onset of symptoms and after blood-clotting had begun and after blood-clotting drugs had been administered. The two trials were as dissimilar as apples and oranges, yet the debate over magnesium's efficacy still rages. Since the LIMIT and ISIS studies, several smaller trials have shown even greater recovery from heart attacks using intravenous magnesium, including a trial of 200 people with a 74 percent lower death rate.[27]

Dr. Michael Shechter is a brilliant young magnesium researcher who in his numerous recent clinical trials has proven the benefits of magnesium in treating heart disease. His clinical trials begun in 2000 and continued every year since maintain that magnesium is a viable and necessary treatment for people with heart disease in spite of the ISIS trial and another trial called MAGIC suggesting that it does not.[28, 29, 30, 31, 32, 33]

Pharmaceutical companies, who want to promote their own drug therapies, cite the ISIS trial as proof that magnesium sulfate doesn't work; supporters of magnesium cite the LIMIT trial as proof that it does. Your doctor may be influenced by the ISIS trial and think magnesium is not an important option in your care. But cardiologists who are looking for alternatives to drug therapy and to its many side effects, and who read studies thoroughly, are using magnesium successfully. To help you find these doctors, there is a list in the Resources section of complementary medicine associations whose doctors study alternatives to the drug-based medicine they learned in medical school. You can also check www.carolyn.dean.com, as I keep abreast of the latest magnesium research.

Because one of the major side effects of heart medications, especially diuretics, is magnesium deficiency, it is vital that magnesium be tested with a red blood cell magnesium test or the EXATest and supplemented in heart patients who are on medication. The dosage ranges from 6 to 10 mg/kg/day (300–1,000 mg per day), but this should be taken only under a doctor's supervision if you are on any other heart medications. See page 115 for magnesium dosage.

SPASTIC HEART

Between 40 and 60 percent of people who suffer sudden heart attacks may actually have no arterial blockage or history of irregular heartbeats.[34] Two suspected causes are spasms in the coronary arteries and the occurrence of a severe heart rhythm disturbance, such as atrial fibrillation. Both of these conditions can be caused by a deficiency of magnesium. Low magnesium makes the heart muscle hyperirritable, leading to the development of a rhythm disturbance that can't be stopped without emergency medical intervention. An astute physician recognizes the possibility of magnesium deficiency and immediately gives magnesium intravenously, as in the LIMIT trial. Rapid heartbeat or atrial tachycardia, premature beats, and atrial fibrillation have all responded to treatment with IV magnesium.[35, 36, 37]

The most common time for the onset of heart attacks is around 9 A.M. on Mondays as people gird themselves for another long workweek.[38] As mentioned earlier, people who suffer from spasm-induced angina attacks most often experience them at the same time each day, usually in the morning and late afternoon, when magnesium levels are at their lowest. The morning deficiency is likely the result of overnight fasting and the loss of magnesium through the urine. Deficiency in the afternoon may be caused by depletion of magnesium induced by the stress of the day and not yet replenished by the evening meal. In view of this, it seems reasonable that people with angina, heart spasms, hypertension, or heart disease should consult with their doctors and take a red blood cell magnesium test or EXATest; if it shows a deficiency, they should take at least 125 mg of magnesium taurate three times each day— before breakfast, at 2 P.M., and before going to bed.

ARRHYTHMIA

Magnesium's ability to neutralize the heart-damaging effects of catecholamines (the products of stress-induced adrenaline and cortisol) is the miracle that can prevent many of the side effects of acute heart attack such as arrhythmia.[39] Magnesium deficiency contributes to abnormal heart rhythms, possibly because magnesium is responsible for maintaining normal potassium and sodium concentrations inside heart muscle cells. A balance of potassium, sodium, calcium, and magnesium allows for normal heart muscle contraction and maintains normal heartbeat. A central pacemaker within the heart muscle creates a normal pumping action that travels across the heart; cardiac arrhythmia occurs when other, less suitable areas of the heart are forced to assume the role of the central pacemaker when it becomes damaged or irritated by lack of oxygen due to blocked blood vessels, caused by drugs (including caffeine), hormonal imbalance, or deficiency of magnesium. These new pacemakers are even more sensitive to magnesium deficiency but are responsive to magnesium therapy, which has been successfully used for over sixty years.[40]

Magnesium is also an accepted treatment for ventricular arrhythmias,[41, 42] congestive heart failure where the heart is weak and unable to empty after each heartbeat,[43, 44] and before and after heart surgery, including coronary bypass grafting.[45, 46, 47] All these studies indicate that the frequency of ventricular arrhythmias is reduced by administration of intra-venous magnesium and support an early high-dose adminis-tration of intravenous magnesium in the wake of myocardial infarction.

MITRAL VALVE PROLAPSE

Magnesium deficiency has been implicated in mitral valve prolapse (MVP), a disorder in which the mitral valve fails to completely close off one of the heart chambers during heart contraction. It is also called floppy valve syndrome. Blood rushing through the open valve can be heard as a heart mur-mur with a stethoscope. When cardiac ultrasound became more commonplace, the diagnosis of MVP escalated, espe-cially in young women. There is no allopathic treatment for the condition, and in mild and even moderate cases it doesn't cause any symptoms. However, patients are usually warned that they should take antibiotics when having dental work done, to prevent the possibility of bacteria from the gums being picked up in the bloodstream and lodging on the pro-lapsed valve, causing infection. This is a very rare occurrence and some doctors disapprove of this overuse of antibiotics, but it remains a potential liability threat to dentists who don't warn their patients.

Dr. Melvyn Werbach, author of *Nutritional Influences on Disease,* believes that MVP is overdiagnosed and also maintains that it is a magnesium deficiency disease that is well treated by magnesium. The valves of the heart are pulled tight by muscles, which, like any other muscle in the body, depend on magnesium for proper functioning. The mitral valve prolapses because excess calcium relative to magnesium causes it to spasm. Dr. Mildred Seelig reports that low magnesium levels have been found in as many as 85 percent of MVP patients.[48] Sixty percent of 141 individuals with strongly symptomatic

MVP had low magnesium levels, compared to only 5 percent of the control group. Magnesium supplementation given for five weeks reduced the symptoms of chest pain, palpitation, anxiety, low energy, faintness, and difficulty breathing by about 50 percent in this group.[49]

CHELATION THERAPY

Even alternative medicine can make more use of magnesium. Chelation therapy is an intravenous treatment with a chemical called EDTA that pulls out excess calcium from the plaque built up on the arterial walls. It would be much more convenient to use magnesium as part of an oral chelation protocol preventively, to keep calcium from building up in the first place, because balanced amounts of magnesium keep calcium dissolved in the blood and unable to deposit in arterial plaque or kidney stones and gallstones. When intravenous EDTA is used, however, generous amounts of magnesium are usually given as well.

SUPPLEMENTS FOR HEART DISEASE

Magnesium taurate: 125 mg four times per day
Coenzyme Q_{10}: 30 mg three times a day
Bromelain: 500 mg three times a day between meals
Vitamin E as mixed tocopherols: 400 IU twice a day
Crategus tincture: 20 drops two or three times a day
Rutin or quercetin (bioflavonoids): 500 mg daily
Biotin: 5 mg daily

For atherosclerosis add:

Niacin (vitamin B_3): 100 mg three times a day, working up to 6 g daily. Do not use time-release niacin, which has been associated with liver damage. Niacinamide (which does not cause flushing) is not effective for lowering cholesterol.
Folic acid: 800 mcg daily

Vitamin B$_6$: 50 mg daily
Vitamin B complex: 50 mg per day
Vitamin C: 1,000 mg three times a day
Vitamin D: 1,000 IU or 20 minutes in the sun daily (acts as an anti-inflammatory)
Calcium citrate: 500 mg daily (especially aids hypertension). Should be balanced with 750 mg of magnesium to keep it from depositing in arterial plaque.

DIET FOR HEART DISEASE

A good diet is based on free-range chicken, fish (such as wild salmon, which is low in mercury), whole grains, legumes, fruit, and vegetables. Therapeutic foods high in magnesium should be included: garlic, onions, nuts, seeds, wheat germ, and sprouts. Don't fall into the trap of blaming cholesterol above all else. Remember, using margarine is not the answer to heart disease. The proper dietary fats for human consumption are butter, olive oil, flaxseed oil, sesame oil, and coconut oil. The diet for all forms of heart disease should exclude alcohol, coffee, white sugar, white flour, fried foods, and trans fatty acids (found in margarine and in baked, fried, and processed foods). Also read *The Yeast Connection and Women's Health* (Crook and Dean, 2005) and *IBS for Dummies* (Dean and Wheeler, 2005).

CHAPTER EIGHT

═══

OBESITY, SYNDROME X, AND DIABETES

Obesity, syndrome X, and diabetes are part of a continuum of illness that may progress to heart disease if not headed off by good diet, supplements, exercise, and stress reduction. They are not really separate diseases, as we may think, and underlying all this misery we find magnesium deficiency. In fact, there has been a recent addition to our medical vocabulary—it's *diabesity*, a recognition that if someone is about thirty pounds overweight for more than a decade, diabetes will likely occur. People with syndrome X are obese, are on the road to diabetes with insulin resistance, and also have hypertension, elevated cholesterol, and high levels of triglycerides.

> ### THREE THINGS YOU NEED TO KNOW
> ### ABOUT MAGNESIUM AND OBESITY
>
> 1. Magnesium helps the body digest, absorb, and utilize proteins, fats, and carbohydrates.
> 2. Magnesium is necessary for insulin to open cell membranes for glucose.
> 3. Magnesium helps prevent obesity genes from expressing themselves.

THE WEIGHT CONNECTION

Magnesium and the B-complex vitamins are energy nutrients: they activate enzymes that control digestion, absorption, and the utilization of proteins, fats, and carbohydrates. Lack of these necessary energy nutrients causes improper utilization of food, leading to such far-ranging symptoms as hypoglycemia, anxiety, and obesity.

Food craving and overeating can be simply a desire to continue eating past fullness because the body is, in fact, craving nutrients that are missing from processed food. You continue to eat empty calories that pack on the pounds but get you no further ahead in your nutrient requirements.

Magnesium is also necessary in the chemical reaction that allows insulin to usher glucose into cells, where glucose is involved in making energy for the body. If there is not enough magnesium to do this job, both insulin and glucose become elevated. The excess glucose gets stored as fat and contributes to obesity. Having excess insulin puts you on the road toward diabetes.

The connection between stress and obesity cannot be overlooked. The stress chemical cortisol signals a metabolic shutdown that makes losing weight almost impossible. It's as if the body feels it is under an attack such that it must hoard all its resources, including fat stores, and won't let go of them under any inducement. As you read in Chapter 3, magnesium can neutralize the effects of stress.

OBESITY, MORE THAN BAD GENES

The public has been told that obesity is inherited, which makes people think they don't have a hand in creating this problem and can continue their bad habits and blame their genes. Animal experiments show, however, that if a mouse with an obesity gene is deprived of B vitamins, the obesity will be expressed. But if it is fed plenty of B vitamins, it will remain thin. The process of metabolizing B vitamins is called methylation, and magnesium is necessary for one of the most important steps. Every metabolic function in the body requires vitamins and minerals—without them, symptoms develop. Therefore, the first step in treating nonspecific symptoms is diet and dietary supplements, not drugs.

It is also important to note that many of the weight loss diets that people subject themselves to are often deficient in magnesium. The better solution would be to follow the Magnesium Eating Plan outlined in Chapter 17.

ABDOMINAL OBESITY

Gaining weight around your middle is related to magnesium deficiency and an inability to properly utilize insulin. It also sets the stage for syndrome X. You only need a tape measure to diagnose a predisposition to syndrome X—a waist size above 40 inches in men and above 35 in women puts you at risk.

In their book *The Magnesium Factor,* authors Mildred Seelig, M.D., and Andrea Rosanoff, Ph.D., take note of research showing that over half the insulin in the bloodstream is directed at abdominal tissue. They theorize that as more and more insulin is produced to deal with a high-sugar diet, abdominal girth increases to process the extra insulin.

SYNDROME X

The term "syndrome X" describes a set of conditions that many believe is just another fancy name for the consequences of long-standing nutritional deficiency, especially magnesium deficiency. The long list includes high cholesterol and hypertension, detailed in Chapter 6, and obesity. It also encompasses elevated triglycerides and elevated uric acid. High triglycerides are usually found when cholesterol is elevated but most often when someone has a high-sugar diet, such as from drinking sodas daily and eating cakes and pastries. High uric acid is due to incomplete breakdown of protein from lack of B vitamins and digestive enzymes. This complex collectively appears to be caused by disturbed insulin metabolism (initiated by magnesium deficiency), called insulin resistance, and eventually can lead to diabetes, angina, and heart attack.

As previously noted, magnesium is required in the metabolic pathways that allow insulin to usher glucose into cells, where glucose participates in making energy for the body. If magnesium is deficient, the doorway into the cells does not open to glucose, resulting in the following cascade of events:

1. Glucose levels become elevated.
2. Glucose is stored as fat and leads to obesity.
3. Elevated glucose leads to diabetes.
4. Obesity puts a strain on the heart.
5. Excess glucose becomes attached to certain proteins (glycated), leading to kidney damage, neuropathy, blindness, and other diabetic complications.

6. Insulin-resistant cells don't allow magnesium into the cells.
7. Further magnesium deficiency leads to hypertension.
8. Magnesium deficiency leads to cholesterol buildup, and both these conditions are implicated in heart disease.

Syndrome X, according to Dr. Gerald Reaven, who coined the term, may be responsible for a large percentage of the heart and artery disease that occurs today. Unquestionably, magnesium deficiency is a major factor in the origins of each of its signs and symptoms, from elevated triglycerides and obesity to disturbed insulin metabolism.[1, 2]

INSULIN RESISTANCE

Insulin's job is to open up sites on cell membranes to allow the influx of glucose, a cell's source of fuel. Cells that no longer respond to the advances of insulin and refuse the entry of glucose are called insulin-resistant. As a result, blood glucose levels rise and the body produces more and more insulin, to no avail. Glucose and insulin rampage throughout the body, causing tissue damage that results in overuse and wasting of magnesium, an increased risk of heart disease, and adult-onset diabetes. One of the major reasons the cells don't respond to insulin is lack of magnesium.[3] Some studies show that chronic insulin resistance in patients with type II diabetes is associated with a reduction of magnesium; magnesium is necessary to allow glucose to enter cells.[4] Additional studies confirm that when insulin is released from the pancreas, magnesium in the cell normally responds and opens the cell to allow entry of glucose, but in the case of magnesium deficiency combined with insulin resistance the normal mechanisms just don't work.[5] However, the higher the levels of magnesium in the body, the greater the sensitivity of the cells to insulin and the possibility of reversing the problem.[6]

CARDIOVASCULAR METABOLIC SYNDROME (CVMS)

Dr. Larry Resnick of Cornell University, involved in heart and magnesium research for over twenty years, has another name for syndrome X. He calls it cardiovascular metabolic syndrome (CVMS), and Dr. Resnick is closer to the truth about this condition when he says it is characterized by a high calcium-to-magnesium ratio. (Remember, too much calcium automatically creates a magnesium deficiency.)[7] Americans in general have a high calcium-to-magnesium ratio in their diet and consequently in their bodies. Finland, which has the highest incidence of heart attack in middle-aged men in the world, also has a high calcium-to-magnesium ratio in the diet. The U.S. ratio in this study is said to be 3.5:1, Finland's 4:1.[8] (With our dietary emphasis on a high calcium intake without sufficient magnesium, according to magnesium expert Dr. Mildred Seelig, we will soon be faced with a 6:1 ratio in our population.) Although the conventional recommended dietary ratio of calcium to magnesium is 2:1, in order to offset the deficiency that many people with syndrome X already have, it may be necessary to ingest one part calcium to one part magnesium in supplement form.

MAGNESIUM DEFICIENCY AND METABOLIC SYNDROME X

According to Dr. Resnick, syndrome X is caused not by chronically elevated insulin levels but by a low level of magnesium ions—because insufficient magnesium is the cause of insulin resistance in the first place.[9] As stated, insulin opens the cells to glucose only if the cells have sufficient amounts of magnesium, and without magnesium, insulin resistance occurs. Studies clearly show that animals deprived of dietary magnesium develop insulin resistance, and the human population has the same risk.[10] Some researchers conclude that hypertension and insulin resistance may just be different expressions of deficient levels of cellular magnesium.[11] The various conditions that make up syndrome X, CVMS, or metabolic syndrome X, its most recent designation, all have similar origins in magnesium deficiency.

The magnesium deficiency in syndrome X comes from a combination of our magnesium-deficient diet and the well-documented loss of magnesium in the urine caused by elevated insulin. A vicious cycle creates further magnesium losses, causing more syndrome X symptoms. In a fifteen-year study of 5,000 young adults, it was found that the more magnesium in the diet or taken as supplements, the lower the likelihood of developing metabolic syndrome.[12]

The cornerstone of both prevention and treatment of syndrome X, along with diet, is to restore magnesium to normal levels. Unfortunately, for many, the ravages of diabetes, hypertension, and high cholesterol have taken their toll, but even then, magnesium taken along with medications can play a beneficial role in controlling and reducing symptoms.[13, 14]

DIABETES

Diabetes is the seventh-leading cause of death in this country. There are 16 million diabetics in the United States, with the numbers increasing dramatically as the population gets older and as more young people succumb to a high-sugar diet. There are two main types of diabetes. About 10 percent of diabetics are labeled type I and are dependent on insulin. Type I diabetes usually develops in children; they may have suffered a viral infection of the pancreas, resulting in impaired or absent insulin production, and require insulin injections to replace their loss. Type II or adult-onset diabetics tend to be non-insulin-dependent, overweight, and between fifty and seventy years old at onset. In type II diabetes, insulin is readily available—in fact, it is usually elevated—but the cells of the body appear to be resistant to it. Insulin is unable to do its job of opening up the cell membrane to allow the passage of glucose into the cell to create energy.

THREE THINGS YOU NEED TO KNOW
ABOUT MAGNESIUM AND DIABETES

1. Magnesium deficiency may be an independent predictor of diabetes.
2. Diabetics both need more magnesium and lose more than most people.
3. Magnesium is necessary for the production, function, and transport of insulin.

A third type of diabetes, gestational diabetes, is usually short-lived. This glucose intolerance may have been present but undetected before pregnancy but usually develops due to the stresses of pregnancy. Ionic magnesium testing demonstrates the presence of magnesium depletion in pregnancy itself and to a greater extent in gestational diabetes. However, ionic magnesium testing remains available only as a research tool; the next best option is a red blood cell magnesium test or an EXATest, either of which is vitally important in diagnosing magnesium deficiency in gestational diabetes. (See Resources for more information.) Magnesium depletion, or relative calcium excess, may predispose women to vascular complications of pregnancy and needs to be addressed.[15] Intervention with magnesium supplements can greatly improve the outcome for both mother and baby.

The signs and symptoms of diabetes are polydipsia (excessive thirst), polyuria (excessive urination), and polyphagia (excessive eating). In type I diabetes, weight loss may be the first sign, but type II diabetics are usually overweight. The excessive urination carries both sugar and magnesium out of the body. The excessive sugar, excreted through the urine and sweat, provides food for the yeast organism *Candida albicans*, resulting in rashes on the skin (especially under the breasts and in the groin area), yeast vaginitis in women, and yeast discharge in men.

Common complications of diabetes include nerve damage, called diabetic neuropathy, which mostly affects the feet, with symptoms of numbness, tingling, burning, and pain; atherosclerosis and heart attacks; damage to small blood vessels in the eyes and kidneys, causing vision loss (diabetes is the leading cause of blindness in the United States) and kidney disease; diabetic foot ulcers, with increased susceptibility to infection, gangrene, and amputation; and impotence in men. All these complications relate to magnesium deficiency and demonstrate the need for sensitive magnesium testing and magnesium supplementation for diabetes.[16]

One diabetic complication that may not be obvious is the tendency for doctors to put diabetics on statin medication. Because diabetes and elevated cholesterol are associated, drug companies promote the use of statins, presumably as a preventive measure. This, however, may not be such a good idea for people who are already suffering symptoms of magnesium deficiency.

Low magnesium levels serve as a relatively new marker for diabetes, occurring in up to 40 percent of diabetic patients.[17, 18, 19] However, if some doctors are skeptical, no one can deny the results from three of the largest studies on the incidence of diseases, the Harvard Nurses' Health Study of 85,000 women, the 43,000 men in the Health Professionals

Follow-Up Study, and another 40,000 women in the Iowa Women's Health Study. All three studies observed that people with the highest levels of the mineral magnesium in their diets have the lowest risk for developing diabetes. It's important that this information be promoted more widely.

DIABETIC COMPLICATIONS AND MAGNESIUM

Lack of magnesium increases the risk of cardiovascular disease, eye symptoms, and nerve damage in diabetics, whereas supplementation can prevent them.[20, 21, 22] Magnesium is a necessary cofactor in the production of energy from sugar stores in the muscles and liver. Most important for diabetics, insulin's main job requires magnesium; without magnesium, insulin is not properly secreted from the pancreas, and what does get into the bloodstream doesn't work correctly. At the cell level, magnesium is required to open pathways into the cell for the entrance of blood sugar. If magnesium is in short supply, sugar stays in the bloodstream, and as it becomes elevated, symptoms of diabetes appear. One of the symptoms of diabetes is copious urination—magnesium levels are elevated in diabetic urine, which means greater losses and more symptoms in a vicious cycle of depletion.

Studies show that even moderate improvement of blood sugar control in patients with type I diabetes seems to reduce the loss of magnesium, increase serum HDL cholesterol (the "good" cholesterol), and decrease serum triglycerides. These reductions in magnesium loss and serum triglycerides and the elevation of good cholesterol may reduce the risk of developing cardiovascular disease in patients with type I diabetes.[23]

DIABETES AND CHILDREN

In his book *Transdermal Magnesium Therapy*, Mark Sircus, O.M.D., asks the question, "Is a lack of magnesium related to type 2 diabetes in obese children?" He answers by reporting on a study by Dr. Huerta showing that magnesium deficiency is associated with insulin resistance in obese children. When checking the dietary intake of magnesium, Dr. Huerta and her colleagues found that 55 percent of obese children did not get enough magnesium from the foods they ate, compared with only 27 percent of nonobese children.

HOW DID WE BECOME A NATION OF DIABETICS?

In non-Western cultures, where most traditional diets are composed largely of unprocessed foods and are low in sugar, it takes only one generation of people eating a more typical Western diet high in sugar and refined flour to develop diabetes. This is true of people around the world, from the Inuit to secluded African peoples. The immediate advice given to a newly diagnosed diabetic is to stop eating sugar and other refined carbohydrates. It is only common sense that avoiding these unhealthy nonfoods as a preventive measure could greatly reduce the incidence of diabetes, yet the medical community has been slow to promote this idea.

Partly as a result, both obesity and type II diabetes are on the rise in children. In the last decade, soft drink consumption has almost doubled among kids, adding an average of 15 to 20 extra teaspoon of sugar a day just from soda and other sugared drinks. These all-too-popular beverages account for more than a quarter of all drinks consumed in the United States. More than 15 billion gallons were sold in 2000.[24] A 2001 report in the prestigious medical journal *The Lancet* revealed that each additional soft drink a day gives a child a 60 percent greater chance of becoming obese.[25] Dr. France Bellisle, of France's Institute of Health and Medical Research, said the study provided convincing new evidence about the relationship between sugar and weight gain in children. It is unfortunate that it has taken so long for the *first* study on sugar and weight gain to be funded and published—so many children and adults are already addicted to sugar, and there is no turning back. Surprisingly, not until diabetes strikes does any medical body recommend cutting back on sugar intake.

LABORATORY FINDINGS IN DIABETES

- Blood glucose greater than or equal to 200 mg/dl (11.1 mmol/L) two hours after an oral dose of 75 g of glucose dissolved in water
- Incidental blood glucose greater than or equal to 200 mg/dl (11.1 mmol/L) in someone with signs and symptoms of diabetes
- High cholesterol
- Low magnesium ions

We know from other important research that obese children develop insulin resistance, a precursor to diabetes, fifty-three times more frequently than normal kids. The number of obese children in the United States doubled between 1980 and 1994; today 24 percent of kids are obese. Recently there has been a 70 percent rise in diabetes in thirty-year-olds, and the trend shows no sign of abating.

As a nation, we eat 140 pounds of sugar per year per person, so it is no wonder that more and more people are developing symptoms of diabetes and insulin resistance and suffering from magnesium deficiency. Even more shocking are studies in both animals and healthy adults that demonstrate a greatly depressed immune response to infection that lasts for more than five hours after the ingestion of 20 tsp of sugar.[26, 27, 28] Part of the danger with sugar is that you may not even realize how much you are ingesting. On ingredient labels, the measurements are given in grams, even though most Americans think in teaspoons, so our eyes may not even register the amounts. People are stunned when told there are 8 to 10 tsp of sugar in an ordinary soda (1 tsp of sugar is equivalent to 4.2 g). Even more shocking is the amount of sugar found in most single servings of sweetened yogurt, which most people think of as a health food.

Sugar overload can cause magnesium deficiency in several ways. Processed sugar is devoid of vitamins and minerals, leaving empty calories that provide no valuable nutrients. Nutritional research reported by Dr. Abram Hoffer (the originator, with Linus Pauling, of orthomolecular medicine) shows that the refining of sugar removes 93 percent of chromium, 89 percent of manganese, 98 percent of cobalt, 83 percent of copper, 98 percent of zinc, and 98 percent of magnesium. All these minerals are essential to life. In addition, the body has to tap into its own reserves of minerals and vitamins to ensure sugar's digestion.

Inability to utilize sugar results in the formation of toxic products such as pyruvic acid and other abnormal sugars that accumulate in the brain, nervous system, and red blood cells, where they interfere with cell respiration and hasten degenerative disease. Adding sugar to the diet produces an excessively acid condition in the body; to neutralize it the body has to draw upon its stores of the alkaline minerals calcium, magnesium, and potassium. If the acidic condition is severe, calcium and magnesium will even be taken from the bones and teeth, which leads to decay, softening, and ultimately osteoporosis. In summary, magnesium plays a pivotal role in the secretion and function of insulin; without it, diabetes is inevitable. Measurable magnesium deficiency is common in diabetes and in many of its complications, including heart disease, eye damage, high blood pressure, and obesity. When the treatment of diabetes includes magnesium, these problems are prevented or minimized.[29] And we do know that magnesium-rich water in certain communities confers a protective effect against the disease.[30, 31] Magnesium supplementation improves insulin response, improves glucose tolerance, and reduces the stickiness of red blood cell membranes. Magnesium also seems to be essential in the treatment of peripheral vascular disease associated with diabetes.[32] With long-term damage, however, many symptoms may be irreversible, even with adequate magnesium and associated nutrients.

DIET FOR DIABETES

The proper diet for the prevention and treatment of diabetes includes frequent small meals of protein (fish—especially wild salmon, to avoid mercury—and free-range chicken and meat) and complex carbohydrates (whole grains, legumes, and vegetables), as well as the avoidance of simple sugars and white flour. Stevia, from the leaves of a plant that grows in South America, is the best sweetener to use. You can find it in health food stores. Don't use the sugar substitute aspartame, which can worsen blood sugar control and cause weight gain, headaches, nerve damage, and eye damage, because it is made partly from wood alcohol, which breaks down to formaldehyde.[33] Fiber from oat bran, flaxseed, and apples has a positive effect on keeping blood sugar balanced. Also read *The Yeast Connection and Women's Health* (Crook and Dean, 2005) and *IBS for Dummies* (Dean and Wheeler, 2005).

Alternative medicine practitioners also suggest identifying

any existing food allergies by eliminating likely suspects (dairy, wheat, corn) from the diet for several days and then eating several meals of one of the suspected foods in one day or doing a blood test or finger stick for glucose. (*Warning:* do not eat several meals consisting of foods to which you have reacted strongly in the past. Simply keep avoiding them.) If the blood sugar is elevated after eating a particular food, it may be wise to avoid that food and find replacements that do not elevate the blood sugar.

SUPPLEMENTS FOR DIABETES

Magnesium taurate: 125 mg three or four times per day
Vitamin E as mixed tocopherols: 400 IU twice a day
Rutin or quercetin (bioflavonoids): 500 mg daily
Folic acid: 800 mcg daily
Vitamin B_6: 50 mg daily
Vitamin B complex: 50 mg per day
Vitamin C: 1,000 mg three times a day
Vitamin D: 1,000 IU or 20 minutes in the sun daily
Calcium citrate: 500 mg daily
Chromium: chromium picolinate, 500 mcg daily, alternating with brewer's yeast, 1 tbsp three times a day (contains glucose tolerance factor [GTF], which balances blood sugar), or specialized chromium (GTF), 200 mcg twice per day
Zinc picolinate: 15 mg daily
Copper: 2–4 mg daily
Selenium: 200 mcg daily
Manganese: 5 mg daily
Vanadium: 15 mg daily
Omega-3 fatty acids: 5 g daily
Garlic: one or two cloves daily

CHAPTER NINE

PMS, DYSMENORRHEA, AND POLYCYSTIC OVARIAN SYNDROME

THREE THINGS YOU NEED TO KNOW ABOUT MAGNESIUM AND PMS

1. Chocolate, which some women have a craving for when they're premenstrual, contains high amounts of magnesium, but the added sugar and fat make it far less desirable as a food.
2. The patent for Prozac has run out, so it has been patented under a new name, Serafem, for PMS. PMS is not caused by a Serafem deficiency, but magnesium deficiency can cause some forms of PMS.
3. Magnesium is a safe treatment for PMS and PMS headaches.

Maureen didn't know what came over her every month, but she would get anxious and irritable and go on a chocolate binge. She tried to keep it to herself, but lately the other women at work had begun to make not-so-subtle comments and tease her about her "evil twin." Then Anna sat with her over lunch one day and told her about a support group she was leading for women with premenstrual syndrome. One of their self-help methods was to keep a journal of symptoms. Maureen's journal for the next couple of months clearly showed that her symptoms of anxiety, fluid retention, sugar and chocolate cravings, mood swings, irritability, bloating, edema, headache, and sore breasts escalated before her period and lifted the minute her period began.

Taking magnesium supplements may be the solution for PMS, advises Melvyn Werbach, M.D. Recent studies showed that of 192 women taking 400 mg of magnesium daily for PMS, 95 percent experienced less breast pain and had less weight gain, 89 percent suffered less nervous tension, and 43 percent had fewer headaches. (Dr. Werbach and several other researchers also advise that women should take 50 mg of vitamin B_6 daily with the magnesium to assist in magnesium absorption.)[1] Red blood cell magnesium tests show low levels of magnesium in women with PMS.[2] Even serum magnesium levels, which are low only when there is a severe magnesium deficiency, diminished significantly in the premenstrual week in a group of forty women.[3] In a small trial of thirty-two women, oral magnesium was found to be an effective treatment of premenstrual symptoms related to mood changes.[4] Treatment with magnesium eases headaches, sugar cravings, low blood sugar, and dizziness related to PMS.[5, 6]

In another innovative research study, magnesium ion levels were taken at several times during normal menstrual cycles to determine magnesium and calcium levels in relation to menstrual phases.[7] There was a comparatively high magnesium ion level in the first week after the onset of the period, a statistically significant decrease in magnesium ions around the time of ovulation, and a large decrease in magnesium ions and serum magnesium when the serum progesterone concentration peaked in the third week. There was also a significant increase in the serum calcium-to-magnesium ratio both at the time of ovulation and in the fourth week after the onset of the period. That calcium-to-magnesium imbalance can cause premenstrual symptoms during the last week of the menstrual cycle. The good news is that you can take care of it easily by taking the right amounts of calcium and magnesium. For most women this translates into equal amounts of calcium and magnesium, 600–1,000 mg of each a day in divided doses. However, if you eat dairy, greens, and whole grains, you will need even less calcium—about 300 mg less.

An elegant study demonstrates that estrogen and progesterone, the female sex hormones, influence magnesium ion levels in the body, which may help explain why magnesium relieves symptoms of PMS, including migraine, bloating, and edema.[8] Exposure of cultured smooth muscle cells from brain blood vessels to a low concentration of estrogen did not interfere with the level of magnesium ions. However, exposure to increased concentrations of estrogen induced significant loss of magnesium ions; at the highest concentration, the level of magnesium ions decreased approximately 30 percent in comparison with controls. Exposure of the cultured cells to a low concentration of progesterone resulted in an increased level of magnesium ions. However, when these cells were exposed to higher concentrations of progesterone, cellular levels of magnesium ions decreased significantly. The higher the estrogen or progesterone concentration, the lower the levels of magnesium ions.

The data in this experiment indicate that the normally low concentrations of the female sex hormones, estrogen and progesterone, help cerebral vascular smooth muscle cells sustain normal concentrations of magnesium ions, which are beneficial to vascular function, whereas high levels of estrogen and progesterone significantly deplete magnesium ions, possibly resulting in cerebral vessel spasms and reduced cerebral blood flow—and thus leading to premenstrual syndrome and migraine and possible stroke risk. These findings help to explain why more women than men suffer migraines and why migraines occur more frequently in the second half of the menstrual cycle, when estrogen and progesterone are both elevated.

Guy Abraham, M.D., a retired obstetrician and gynecologist, is a widely published author who has pursued major research on premenstrual syndrome. Dr. Abraham identifies four types of PMS, each of which has distinct characteristics related to hormonal fluctuations.

1. PMS-A (anxiety), with symptoms of mood swings, nervous tension, irritability, anxiety. Related to high estrogen, low progesterone.
2. PMS-C (craving), with symptoms of increased appetite, headache, fatigue, dizziness, fainting, palpitations. Related to increased carbohydrate intake and decreased prostaglandin E1–type foods (from fish, nuts, seeds).
3. PMS-D (depression), with symptoms of depression, crying, forgetfulness, confusion, insomnia. Related to low estrogen, high progesterone, elevated male hormone with excess hair growth.
4. PMS-H (hyperhydration), with symptoms of fluid retention, weight gain, swollen extremities, breast tenderness, abdominal bloating. Related to excess aldosterone (a kidney hormone that causes fluid retention).

Maureen had symptoms from three of the four groups. Her successful treatment involved balancing hormones and replacing deficient nutrients. She began to take a daily tablespoon of flaxseed oil, which contains omega-3 essential fatty acids, along with magnesium, vitamin B_6, and calcium. Essential fatty acids are necessary building blocks for hormone production as long as they have magnesium and B vitamins as cofactors.

PMS AND YOUR DIET

A fascinating diet review shows that women suffering from PMS followed diets that were

275 percent higher in refined sugar

79 percent higher in dairy products

78 percent higher in sodium

77 percent lower in magnesium

63 percent higher in refined carbohydrates

53 percent lower in iron

52 percent lower in zinc[9]

Ounce for ounce, chocolate has more magnesium than any other food, and the irresistible urge to consume chocolate is a sure sign of magnesium deficiency. Premenstrual chocolate craving is widespread because magnesium is at its lowest around that time of a woman's menses. The answer is not to eat more chocolate, however, but to increase magnesium intake by eating more nuts, whole grains, seafood, and green vegetables, and by taking magnesium supplements. The chocolate cravings will vanish when there is enough magnesium in the diet.

Other foods to consume in moderation are beef and chicken, which are frequently treated with synthetic hormones. Remember that one type of PMS occurs when there is too much estrogen and too little progesterone in a woman's body. It is possible to end up with too much estrogen stimulation by eating, drinking, or breathing synthetic hormones, pesticides, or other chemical residues that mimic estrogen. The saturated fat and arachidonic acid in meat also suppress progesterone production and cause symptoms of inflammation that worsen PMS and can lead to painful periods. Essential fatty acids—from fish, nuts, and seeds, including flaxseed—are much healthier fats and help prevent PMS, unless you have a magnesium deficiency. Without magnesium, essential fatty acids are not processed properly and are not able to calm the irritability and inflammation of PMS and painful periods. Magnesium deficiency is created by stress, which is common to PMS sufferers. The only solution to this vicious circle is to eat a healthy diet—organic, if possible—and take nutrient supplements that include magnesium.

PMS AND DEPRESSION

Women can get depressed before their period, but PMS is not just depression. Yet PMS is often considered by medical doctors and pharmaceutical companies to be a psychiatric condition suitable for treatment with selective serotonin reuptake inhibitors such as fluoxetine (Prozac, Serafem). But remember that a lack of fluoxetine does not cause PMS symptoms; a lack of magnesium does. The replacement of magnesium in the body will treat PMS and cause no side effects. In fact, it has also been found that magnesium relieves the depression of premenstrual syndrome by positively influencing serotonin activity naturally. Serafem can make no such claim.

TREATMENT FOR PMS

DIET
Increase complex carbohydrates and fiber.
Reduce saturated fats, particularly red meat and dairy.
Eliminate caffeine and alcohol.
Reduce salt intake.
Eliminate sugar.

SUPPLEMENTS FOR PMS

Magnesium citrate: 300–900 mg daily

Vitamin B6: 100 mg three times a day for ten days before the period starts

Vitamin B complex: 50 mg daily

Vitamin E as mixed tocopherols: 400 IU daily

Essential fatty acids: flaxseed oil, 1 tbsp twice per day, or evening primrose oil, 500 mg three times per day

Calcium citrate: 500 mg daily

Milk thistle: 250 mg three times a day, to detox the liver

Progesterone: $1/4$ tsp twice a day rubbed into the skin (rotate among inner thighs, stomach, inner arms). Use natural progesterone cream derived from wild yam to balance excess estrogen. It should contain USP progesterone 450–500 mg/oz. (Before using progesterone cream, have a naturopathic doctor evaluate your hormones by testing levels in your saliva and retest every three to four months to avoid overdosing, which can deplete magnesium.)

DYSMENORRHEA (PAINFUL PERIODS)

Calcium can act like a painkiller and relaxant, but it may accomplish this by driving magnesium out of the cells and into the bloodstream, where it is able to be directed toward ailing tissues to treat pain. So taking calcium can alleviate menstrual cramps in this way—until you become magnesium-depleted. Taking magnesium *before* your period may forestall the pain altogether. A series of European studies with small groups of women who suffered painful periods consistently showed relief of symptoms when they took high doses of magnesium.[10, 11, 12]

A balanced calcium and magnesium supplement (300 mg calcium citrate and 300 mg magnesium citrate, twice per day) helps to ensure adequate levels of both minerals and should be taken preventively (use less calcium if you eat calcium-rich foods such as dairy, greens, and grains). Extra magnesium can also be taken when the pain is at its worst (300 mg once or twice a day for a total of 900–1,200 mg).

Some women find that decreasing their intake of meat before their period helps prevent cramps. What may not be obvious is that when you cut back on meat you have a better chance of eating more magnesium-rich foods that will ease symptoms of painful periods.

POLYCYSTIC OVARIAN SYNDROME

Polycystic ovarian syndrome (PCOS) patients have a high incidence of insulin resistance and glucose intolerance. In a recent telephone consultation, a young woman told me she had been advised to go on diabetes drugs, not because she has diabetes but because she has PCOS and the drugs were supposed to lower her insulin resistance. PCOS patients also tend to be at risk for hypertension, diabetes, and heart disease. Since a low magnesium ion level and a high calcium/magnesium ratio are associated with insulin resistance, cardiovascular problems, diabetes mellitus, and hypertension, a study was done on a group of PCOS patients to determine the effects of magnesium intervention. Significantly lower levels of magnesium ions and serum magnesium and a significantly higher calcium-ion-to-magnesium-ion ratio were found in the PCOS patients compared with the controls, which gave me enough evidence to recommend she speak to her doctor about taking a magnesium citrate supplement of 300 mg twice per day to treat her insulin resistance and possibly her PCOS as well.[13]

≡

CHAPTER TEN

INFERTILITY, PREGNANCY, PREECLAMPSIA, AND CEREBRAL PALSY

Advice passed down through generations of midwives includes giving Epsom salts (magnesium sulfate) throughout pregnancy. Therefore it comes as no surprise that magnesium is an important part of the whole miracle of ushering new life into the world. Conception, pregnancy, and delivery are times when nature, nutrients, and nurturing are the prescription, not drug intervention. I learned this important lesson from the astonishing results in the delivery suite when IV magnesium was used to stop seizures and lower high blood pressure. This powerful yet safe medicine can do much more than we currently allow.

INFERTILITY

The Pottenger Cat Study is very instructive on the absolute requirement for good nutrition in pregnancy. Francis M. Pottenger, M.D., beginning in 1932, ran a ten-year nutritional experiment on several groups of cats. He fed one group heat-processed food and another group raw meat and raw milk. The cats fed cooked food became infertile by the third generation, in contrast to those eating the raw food diet. This simple study underscores the importance not just of magnesium but of all nutrients in producing a viable pregnancy. We know that heating food past the boiling point destroys vitamins and burns off magnesium and enzymes. Most minerals may be left, but the vital balance with other nutrients is ultimately lost.

Dr. Sherry Rogers, a diplomate in family practice, allergy-asthma-immunology, and environmental medicine and a fellow of the American College of Nutrition, says that just as migraines are caused by spasms in the brain arteries, spasms in the fallopian tubes cause infertility. This may explain why so many infertile women get pregnant when they go on a whole-foods diet and take supplements including magnesium.[1] Magnesium is required in higher amounts during pregnancy.[2] So taking it to enhance conception also creates a healthier pregnancy.

It also appears that male infertility is associated with magnesium deficiency. Both magnesium and zinc are found in very significant amounts in seminal fluid. However, infertile men have much lower levels of magnesium, especially when they also have chronic prostatitis or prostate infection.[3]

SEIZURES IN THE DELIVERY SUITE

Marie was not having an easy pregnancy. She had gained too much weight, she had headaches, and her ankles and hands were swollen. She also felt a tightness in her head and shortness of breath. At her eight-month visit to the doctor, her blood pressure was elevated, she had hyperactive reflexes, and her urine showed protein—all symptoms of preeclampsia (also called pregnancy-induced hypertension or toxemia). Preeclampsia occurs in 7 percent of all pregnancies and, according to the Preeclampsia Foundation, is responsible for at least 76,000 maternal deaths worldwide each year. A rapidly progressive condition characterized by high blood pressure, hyperactive reflexes, edema, headaches, changes in vision, and protein in the urine, it can escalate and cause seizures, at which point it is called eclampsia.

Eclampsia is a serious condition that can cause premature labor, premature birth, and cerebral palsy in the newborn. Marie's doctor said that bed rest was the only solution to lower her blood pressure but that if she continued to have high blood pressure around the time of delivery, he would give her intravenous magnesium. Unfortunately, he did not have her current magnesium levels tested. Many researchers and clinicians recommend that pregnant women have a red blood cell magnesium test or EXATest and take 300–600 mg of supplemental magnesium.[4, 5, 6] (Always check with your obstetrician or health care provider before adding any supplement, but know that magnesium has a long history of safety for both mother and child.)

Although magnesium is the treatment of choice for pregnancy-induced hypertension, it could be used more widely. Many researchers suggest that pregnant mothers routinely take magnesium throughout pregnancy to prevent complications during delivery and postpartum, and to help prevent premature births.[7] Clinical trials have demonstrated that mothers supplementing with magnesium oxide have larger, healthier babies and lower rates of preeclampsia, premature labor, sudden infant death, and birth defects, including cerebral palsy.[8] What has become apparent in recent studies, however, is that only 4 percent of magnesium oxide is absorbed and utilized in the body. (In Chapter 18 the various types of magnesium products that are available are listed to help you decide which one is best for you.) Fortunately, Marie consulted a midwife specializing in preeclampsia, who was familiar with the use of magnesium in pregnancy. They checked the label of Marie's prenatal supplement and found that it contained only 150 mg of magnesium; she really needed at least 360 mg just to meet the RDA for pregnant women. The midwife recommended that Marie take a magnesium supplement to give her a total of 400 mg of elemental magnesium per day and that she increase her intake of magnesium-rich foods.

Magnesium sulfate given intravenously for eclampsia has been used successfully for more than seventy-five years.[9] In the 1960s, the advent of new diuretics and anticonvulsant drugs threatened to displace magnesium sulfate. Drug companies continue to run expensive clinical trials to compare their newest antihypertensives and anticonvulsants to magnesium sulfate. Most studies show that magnesium is, in fact, more effective than synthetic medications, decreases both infant and maternal mortality, and is extremely safe. As one researcher remarked, "The significant improvement in fetal outcome with dietary magnesium supports the concept of magnesium supplementation during pregnancy."[10]

On this new regimen, Marie noticed many positive changes. She had less back and neck tension, was no longer constipated (a common side effect of pregnancy), had more energy, and lost her edema and puffiness. Finally, the tightness in her head lessened and her blood pressure began to go down. When she told all this to her obstetrician, he actually apologized for not being more aware of her magnesium status and said it was a good reminder for him to be more diligent about the amount of magnesium in his patients' prenatal supplements.

SIDS

Magnesium deficiency has been implicated in sudden infant death syndrome (SIDS), which has features in common with sudden cardiac death of adults[11] and may be prevented by giving adequate magnesium to the mother and child.[12] An episode of muscular weakness induced by magnesium deficiency could prevent a distressed infant from turning its head when lying facedown and thus result in suffocation.[13]

The triple-risk model for SIDS describes the intersection of three potential risks: (1) a vulnerable newborn who is magnesium-deficient, (2) a critical adjustment and development period in a newborn displaying hyperirritability and unsettled cardiovascular and respiratory control, and (3) an outside stressor such as high-pitched noise, excessive motion or handling, chill, fever, or vaccination. Together, these three risks may trigger a shocklike episode of apnea, unconsciousness, and slow heart rate. Researchers feel that it is likely that a high proportion of SIDS deaths could be prevented by simple oral magnesium supplementation to infants during the first critical weeks and months of life.[14] This could be given in the form of a magnesium citrate or magnesium chloride powder in a bottle of water.

Dr. Jean Durlach, a professor at St. Vincent de Paul Hospital in Paris and president of the International Society for the Development of Research on Magnesium (SDRM), states, "This simple and cheap supplementation with doses of 300 milligrams per day to the mother is ethically justifiable. Furthermore the beneficial effects of magnesium supplementation are well established for the mother, for fetal development, and for the baby at birth." He calls for a large clinical trial of magnesium supplementation in pregnant and breast-feeding women.[15]

CEREBRAL PALSY

Cerebral palsy (CP) can occur when there is a fetal brain hemorrhage during the last stages of pregnancy, either from the mother's high blood pressure or from a lack of oxygen to the developing baby's brain. It can also be caused by low birth weight and prematurity. In cerebral palsy, the brain is damaged in such a way that it is unable to properly direct muscle function. The brain gives the muscles contradictory signals, and as a result, the muscles lock and become spastic or go limp, creating a disabling and incurable condition. Close to half the infants born with CP also have mental handicaps. Very-low-birth-weight babies (less than 1,500 g, or 3.3 lbs) are a hundred times more likely to have disabling CP than infants of average birth weight (3,000–3,500 g); more than 25 percent of all CP occurs in very-low-birth-weight babies. More than half a million Americans suffer from CP, with estimated medical costs of $5 billion a year.

Since there is no treatment for CP, preventing cerebral palsy would be "very desirable indeed," asserts neurologist Karin B. Nelson of the National Institutes of Health in Bethesda, Maryland. Dr. Nelson and her colleagues concluded a groundbreaking study in 1995 showing that very-low-birth-weight babies in four centers in California had a lower incidence of cerebral palsy when their mothers were treated with magnesium sulfate shortly before giving birth.[16] "This intriguing finding means that use of a simple medication could significantly decrease the incidence of cerebral palsy and prevent lifelong disability and suffering for thousands of Americans," said Zach W. Hall, Ph.D., director of the National Institute of Neurological Disorders and Stroke. The researchers calculated that magnesium sulfate reduced the prevalence of cerebral palsy by about 90 percent and reduced the prevalence of mental retardation by about 70 percent. They speculate that magnesium may play a role in brain development and possibly prevent cerebral hemorrhage in preterm infants.

Dr. Diane Schendel found very similar results the following year while studying a population in Atlanta.[17] Those mothers receiving magnesium sulfate delivered infants with a 90 percent lower prevalence of cerebral palsy and a 70 percent lower prevalence of mental retardation. The researchers reported that at one year of age, only 1 out of 113 babies whose mothers received magnesium sulfate developed cerebral palsy. Only two of the babies had mental handicaps. In contrast, 30 of the 405 children whose mothers did not receive magnesium sulfate had cerebral palsy and 22 had handicaps. The investigators speculated that magnesium may prevent fetal brain hemorrhage or block the harmful effects of a diminished oxygen supply to the brain. And for those babies exposed to too much oxygen in an attempt to overcome intrauterine deficits, magnesium protects the lungs.[18] A recent literature review and new research suggest that magnesium chloride might be even more protective for the developing brain than magnesium sulfate.[19, 20]

Beyond magnesium supplementation given to expectant mothers and to newborns, there are certain interventions that can prevent some of the subsequent brain damage to low-birth-weight infants. One is specialized craniosacral massage provided within hours or days of birth by licensed practitioners. Naturopaths can help identify food or airborne allergies that can worsen symptoms, and can recommend a wholesome diet and supplement program. Be warned that many supplements on the shelf contain aspartame, a potent neurotoxin. You should never expose your child to this chemical.

SUPPLEMENTS FOR CHILDREN
WITH CEREBRAL PALSY

Magnesium citrate: 10 mg /kg /day
Zinc: 5 mg per day
Vitamin B complex: 10 mg per day
Vitamin C: 200 mg per day
Bioflavonoids: 100 mg per day
Essential fatty acids: DHA, 1 tsp per day; cod liver oil, 1 tsp per day; flaxseed oil, 1 tsp per day

≡

CHAPTER ELEVEN

OSTEOPOROSIS AND KIDNEY STONES

**THREE THINGS YOU NEED TO KNOW ABOUT
MAGNESIUM, OSTEOPOROSIS,
AND KIDNEY STONES**

---

1. Magnesium is just as important as calcium to prevent and treat osteoporosis.
2. Magnesium keeps calcium dissolved in the blood so it will not form kidney stones.
3. Taking calcium without magnesium for osteoporosis can promote kidney stones.

Muriel wondered how she managed to have soft bones and kidney stones all at the same time. Her recent bone density test showed obvious osteoporosis, yet she was now in the hospital with her third kidney stone attack. A young intern explained that she was losing calcium from her bones, which was being deposited in her kidneys and flushed out as hard, jagged crystals that were excruciatingly painful to pass. The high doses of calcium that she was taking for her osteoporosis were only making matters worse.

Muriel's urologist did an analysis on her kidney stones and told her to stop eating all dairy products and to avoid calcium supplements, but Muriel was very concerned that her osteoporosis would worsen.

When she consulted with me, I was able to explain that there are approximately eighteen nutrients essential for healthy bones, including magnesium, the most important mineral after calcium. Susan Brown, Ph.D., director of the Osteoporosis Education Project in Syracuse, New York, warns that "the use of calcium supplementation in the face of magnesium deficiency can lead to a deposition of calcium in the soft tissue such as the joints, promoting arthritis, or in the kidney, contributing to kidney stones."[1] Dr. Brown recommends a daily dose of only 450 mg of magnesium for the prevention and treatment of osteoporosis.

Women with osteoporosis have lower-than-average levels of magnesium in their diets, according to survey reports. Magnesium deficiency can compromise calcium metabolism and also hinder the body's production of vitamin D, further weakening bones.

Magnesium's role in bone health is multifaceted.

- Adequate levels of magnesium are essential for the absorption and metabolism of calcium.
- Magnesium stimulates a particular hormone, calcitonin, that helps to preserve bone structure and draws calcium out of the blood and soft tissues back into the bones, preventing some forms of arthritis and kidney stones.
- Magnesium suppresses another bone hormone called parathyroid, preventing it from breaking down bone.

- Magnesium converts vitamin D into its active form so that it can help calcium absorption.
- Magnesium is required to activate an enzyme that is necessary to form new bone.
- Magnesium regulates active calcium transport.

With all these roles for magnesium to play, it is no wonder that even a mild deficiency can be a risk factor for osteoporosis. Further, if there is too much calcium in the body, especially from calcium supplementation, as in Muriel's case, magnesium absorption can be greatly impaired, resulting in worsening osteoporosis and the likelihood of kidney stones, arthritis, and heart disease. A chance meeting in a hotel with a woman whose lymphoma worsened immediately after being prescribed 2,500 mg of calcium, but no magnesium, for her osteoporosis made me realize that excess calcium can also deposit in cancerous tumors.

Other factors that are important in the development of osteoporosis include diet, drugs, endocrine imbalance, allergies, vitamin D deficiency, and lack of exercise. A detailed review of the osteoporosis literature shows that chronically low intake of magnesium, vitamin D, boron, and vitamins K, B_{12}, B_6, and folic acid leads to osteoporosis. Similarly, chronically high intake of protein, sodium chloride, alcohol, and caffeine adversely affects bone health.[2, 3] The typical Western diet (high in protein, salt, and refined and processed foods) combined with an increasingly sedentary lifestyle contributes to the increasing incidence of osteoporosis.

Looking at her lifestyle, Muriel saw how much she had contributed to her own condition. She averaged five cups of coffee, three glasses of wine, and twenty cigarettes a day. This was causing calcium and magnesium, and the other nutrients that have to deal with toxins, to be overworked or flushed out of her body. Her diet was mostly nutrient-deficient fast food because she was constantly on the run. Muriel also drank lots of soda, which is high in sugar and phosphorus, both of which cause calcium and magnesium to be eliminated. She also avoided the sun and therefore got little vitamin D.

Instead of becoming discouraged, Muriel was able to look on the bright side. At least now she knew what lifestyle habits she had to change and what supplements to take. Her kidney stones soon became a thing of the past, her overall health dramatically improved, and after two years she had not just stopped losing bone but actually saw an increase in her bone density.

OSTEOPOROSIS MISUNDERSTOOD AND MISTREATED

Osteoporosis is neither a normal nor inevitable consequence of aging: Our bones were designed to last a lifetime. Popular wisdom, however, is that osteoporosis in women is due to a decrease in estrogen levels with age. Doctors therefore rely on estrogen, calcium, and drugs that stimulate bone formation to treat osteoporosis. The National Institutes of Health (NIH) Osteoporosis Prevention, Diagnosis, and Therapy Consensus Statement of 2000 was developed from a conference including eighty experts, but no mention of magnesium deficiency as a causative factor in osteoporosis was made in the final report.[4]

With drug companies funding most of the osteoporosis research, there are no large clinical trials investigating the magnesium connection in bone production. Although I was able to find over 22,000 journal articles on osteoporosis, there were only ten in the past decade that studied the magnesium connection in humans. As long as people are given false hope that there is some magic bullet in the pharmaceutical pipeline that will "cure" osteoporosis, or any other chronic disease, they will ignore the underlying diet- and nutrient-related reasons for their health problems.

The recent report that Fosamax causes jawbone deterioration is evidence that this drug, and likely all bisphosphonates, cause brittle bones. Fosamax destroys osteoclasts, the cells that remodel bone (sculpt the bone as new bone forms). Fosamax is therefore supposed to prevent bone breakdown—but the drug companies did not reckon with the bone-remodeling function of the osteoclast. X-rays of bones under the influence of Fosamax may look like they have more calcium but without the remodeling capacity the bones' internal structure is in disarray, and bones are more brittle, and may actually break more easily.

When you read the scientific literature, there is ample evidence that many nutrients, especially magnesium, play a crucial role in bone development. Much animal research, for example, proves that magnesium depletion alters bone and mineral metabolism, which results in bone loss and osteoporosis.[5, 6] Magnesium deficiency is very common in women with osteoporosis compared to controls.[7]

In one study, postmenopausal women with osteoporosis were able to stop the progression of the disease with 250–750 mg of magnesium daily for two years. Without any other added measures, 8 percent of these women experienced a net increase in bone density.[8] A group of menopausal women given a magnesium hydroxide supplement for two years had fewer fractures and a significant increase in bone density.[9] Another study showed that by taking magnesium lactate (1,500–3,000 mg daily for two years), 65 percent of the women were completely free of pain and had no further degeneration of spinal vertebrae.[10] Magnesium in conjunction with hormonal replacement improved bone density in several groups of women compared to controls.[11, 12] In fact, if you are taking estrogen and have a low magnesium intake, calcium supplementation may increase your risk of thrombosis (blood clotting that can lead to a heart attack).[13]

It is unfortunate that the treatment for osteoporosis has been simplified into the single battle cry "Take calcium." Calcium dominates every discussion about osteoporosis, is used to fortify dozens of foods (including orange juice and cereal), and is a top-selling supplement, but it cannot stand alone. In Chapter 1, we talked about the dance of calcium and magnesium. These minerals work so closely together that the lack of one immediately diminishes the effectiveness of the other. Even though the use of calcium supplementation for the management of osteoporosis has increased significantly in the last decade, scientific studies do not support such large doses after menopause. Soft tissue calcification could be a serious side effect of taking too much calcium.[14]

Osteoporosis is generally a progressive disease, and some say it is incurable, but if you avoid the risk factors that are under your control, take a good range of bone-building nutrients, and exercise, you can halt the condition even if you have the symptoms. Prevention is the best defense, the key elements of which are:

- Eat a balanced, nutrient-rich diet.
- Take supplements of calcium, magnesium, and the various bone support factors.
- Practice a vigorous exercise program throughout life.

DIET FOR OSTEOPOROSIS

A high-protein diet and excess sugar, alcohol, and coffee all rob the body of essential minerals. Prevention in the form of fruit and vegetables containing large amounts of calcium, magnesium, and potassium contributes to maintenance of bone mineral density.[15] Add more vegetables, whole grains, legumes, nuts, and seeds to your diet, and be sure to include some of the magnesium-rich foods listed on pages 255–57.

The foods that are high in calcium are usually abundant in magnesium as well, including nuts and seeds, sardines, bok choy (Chinese cabbage), and broccoli. See the list of foods containing high amounts of calcium on pages 257–58.

SUPPLEMENTS FOR OSTEOPOROSIS

Calcium citrate: 500 mg per day

Magnesium citrate: 300 mg twice a day

Boron: 2 mg daily (involved in vitamin D conversion)

Copper: 1–3 mg daily (for collagen cross-linking)

Manganese: 5–10 mg per day (stimulates the production of mucopolysaccharides, the organic matrix of bone)

Zinc: 10 mg daily (important for bone matrix)

Vitamin A: 20,000 IU daily (forms bone matrix)

Vitamin B_6: 50 mg per day

Folic acid: 800 mcg daily

Vitamin B complex: 50 mg per day

Vitamin C: 1,000 mg per day

Vitamin D: 1,000 IU or 20 minutes in the sun daily (for calcium absorption)

Progesterone for postmenopausal women under the advice of your doctor and after hormonal saliva testing to determine deficiency of progesterone: days 1–25, use ¼ tsp of progesterone cream, rubbed into the skin, twice a day; take a break days 25–31 (make sure the product contains USP progesterone). Test levels every three to six months to prevent progesterone excess.

You can obtain about half your mineral needs from good organic foods. The supplement doses above assume that you are already getting minerals in your diet. If you do not eat a good diet, your mineral supplement amounts should be increased by 50 percent.

KIDNEY STONES

Kidney stones occur when the microscopic debris excreted in the urine becomes too concentrated to pass freely out of the kidneys into the bladder. Kidney stones are quite common in the general population. Risk factors for kidney stones include a history of hypertension, chronic dehydration, and a low dietary intake of magnesium.[16] One percent of autopsies reveal stones in the urinary tract, but most are small enough to pass unnoticed. Up to 15 percent of white men and 6 percent of all women will develop one stone, with recurrence in about half of these people. Approximately one person in a thousand in the United States is hospitalized annually with excruciatingly painful stones trapped in their urinary passages. The pain begins in the lower back and can radiate across the abdomen or into the genitals or the inside of the thigh.

Most kidney stones are made up of calcium phosphate, calcium oxalate, or uric acid. (The kind of stones you have can be determined from an analysis of passed stones.) Calcium stones are seen chiefly in men, often with a family history. Calcium phosphate and calcium oxalate alone are responsible for almost 85 percent of all stones. Uric acid stones make up 5–10 percent of all stones. They are also seen mostly in men, half of whom have gout. The remaining 5 percent are rare stones that can be formed during kidney infections.

Diagnosis is made by urinalysis and X-ray. If there are only a few calcium crystals or small stones, often no treatment may be needed, but pain may be relieved with painkillers and muscle relaxants. Larger stones are treated with surgery or with lithotripsy (the breakdown of the stones into little pieces using special ultrasound machines).

Several factors can be involved in stone formation:

1. Elevated calcium in the urine is caused by a diet high in sugar, fructose, alcohol, coffee, and meat. These acidic foods pull calcium from the bone and excrete it through the kidneys. Calcium supplementation without magnesium also causes elevated calcium in the urine.

2. Higher-than-normal levels of oxalate found in the urine may relate to a high dietary intake of oxalic-acid-containing foods: rhubarb, spinach, chard, raw parsley, chocolate, tea, and coffee, among others. The oxalic acid in them promotes stone formation by binding to calcium, creating insoluble calcium oxalate.

3. Dehydration concentrates calcium and other minerals in the urine. Six to eight glasses of water a day are essential to flush the kidneys properly. Increased sweating and not enough water intake create concentrated urine.

4. Soft drinks containing phosphoric acid encourage kidney stones in some people by pulling calcium out of the bones and depositing it in the kidneys.

5. A diet high in purines (substances found in alcohol, meat, and fish) can cause uric acid kidney stones.

Kidney stones and magnesium deficiency share the same list of causes, including a diet high in sugar, alcohol, oxalates, and coffee. An important animal study shows that a high dietary intake of fructose (from high-fructose corn syrup, used as a sweetener) significantly increases kidney calcification, especially when dietary magnesium is low.[17] The U.S. Department of Agriculture warns that young people, especially, derive too many of their daily calories from the high-fructose corn syrup in sodas and eat few greens, which are rich in magnesium. The phosphoric acid in soft drinks is also punishing to the magnesium in the body and depletes magnesium stores while wearing away bone.[18, 19]

One of magnesium's many jobs is to keep calcium in solution to prevent it from solidifying into crystals; even at times of dehydration, if there is sufficient magnesium, calcium will stay in solution. Magnesium is the pivotal treatment for kidney stones. If you don't have enough magnesium to help dissolve calcium, you will end up with various forms of calcification. This translates into stones, muscle spasms, fibrositis, fibromyalgia, and atherosclerosis (calcification of the arteries).

Dr. George Bunce has clinically proven the relationship between kidney stones and magnesium deficiency.[20] As early as 1964, Bunce reported the benefits of administering a 420 mg dose of magnesium oxide per day to patients who had a history of frequent stone formation.

When there is more calcium than magnesium, kidney stones can form. Let's look at that simple experiment from Chapter 1 again to prove the point. Crush and stir a calcium tablet in 1 oz of water; note how much dissolves and how much is still swirling around in the bottom of the glass. Then add a crushed magnesium tablet, or the contents from a magnesium capsule, to the water and see how much more calcium dissolves. If calcium is dissolved properly in the blood, then it won't form crystals in the kidney.

Several older studies show the benefits of magnesium hydroxide in preventing stone formation. Fifty-five patients with a combined 480 stones in the previous ten years were placed on 200 mg of magnesium hydroxide daily. Patients were followed for two to four years, and only eight patients developed new stones. Of a group of forty-three kidney stone patients who did not receive magnesium, 59 percent developed new kidney stones over a four-year period.[21] An even earlier study using magnesium oxide and vitamin B_6 (a natural diuretic) showed a decrease in stone formation for 149 patients, who went from an average of 1.3 stones per year to 0.1 stones. Patients were followed for between four and a half and six years.[22] In another study, fifty-six patients were given 200 mg of magnesium hydroxide twice per day. At the two-year mark, forty-five were free of kidney stone recurrence; of thirty-four patients not taking magnesium, fifteen had recurrences after two years.[23]

Other studies show that urinary magnesium concentration is abnormally low and urinary calcium concentration is abnormally high in more than 25 percent of patients with kidney stones. Supplemental magnesium intake corrects this abnormality and prevents the recurrence of stones. Other researchers acknowledge that magnesium oxide or magnesium hydroxide therapy causes a considerable lessening of kidney stone recurrence in men and feel that soft tissue calcifications can be stopped and even prevented by magnesium therapy.[24] Magnesium seems to be as effective against stone formation as diuretics, the major drug treatment for kidney stones.[25] Avoidance of calcium, taking diuretics, and mechanical intervention, however, seem to constitute the current allopathic medical approach to kidney stones.

More recent reports indicate that magnesium citrate may be a better choice than either magnesium oxide or magnesium hydroxide because it is better absorbed. Only 4 percent of magnesium oxide finds its way into body tissues. A 2005 review paper notes that while magnesium oxide and magnesium hydroxide had been looked upon favorably for the treatment of kidney stones, magnesium citrate proved to be far superior in double-blind, randomized, placebo-controlled trials, reducing the occurrence of kidney stones by 90 percent.[26]

Epidemiological findings round out the picture of kidney

stone occurrence and its association with low magnesium intake. For example, the disease pattern in Greenland includes a low incidence of heart disease and kidney and urinary tract stones, few cases of diabetes mellitus, and little osteoporosis, all of which may be related to low calcium and high magnesium in Greenlanders' diet.[27]

DIETARY TREATMENT FOR KIDNEY STONES

On a regular basis, drink six to eight glasses of water (with a pH above 7.5) a day; increase intake of green vegetables and fiber (vegetarians have a 40–60 percent decreased risk of stone formation) and foods high in magnesium, such as seeds, vegetables, and whole grains; and decrease consumption of sugar, alcohol, coffee, and meat.

For uric acid kidney stones, decrease consumption of foods high in purine, such as alcohol, anchovies, herring, lentils, meat, mushrooms, organ meats, sardines, seafood, and shellfish. For oxalate stones, decrease consumption of foods high in oxalic acid: red beet tops, black tea, cocoa, cranberry, nuts, parsley, tomatoes, rhubarb, chard, and spinach. The citric acid in lemons, limes, oranges, pineapples, and gooseberries dissolves calcium oxalate and calcium phosphate, preventing stone formation.

SUPPLEMENTS FOR KIDNEY STONES

Magnesium citrate: 300 mg twice per day
Potassium citrate: 300 mg twice per day
Vitamin B_6: 50–100 mg daily

THE RESEARCH CONTINUES

While research identifying magnesium deficiency as a causative factor in heart disease, migraines, and eclampsia is clear-cut, many investigators believe that magnesium also plays an important role in chronic fatigue syndrome, fibromyalgia, environmental illness, and aging. More investigation needs to be done on these conditions to prove that magnesium deficiency is a contributing factor and that magnesium replacement should be part of the treatment protocol. Part Three offers a review of what many clinicians and researchers already know about these conditions and the magnesium connection.

But first, let's look at magnesium through the eyes of John I. Rodale, editor of *Prevention* magazine, who in 1968 wrote *Magnesium: The Nutrient That Could Change*

Your Life (available free online at www.mgwater.com/rodtitle. shtml). Rodale unearthed scientific and clinical research on the use of magnesium in treating infection, polio, epilepsy, alcoholism, prostate inflammation, cancer, and arthritis. Unfortunately, much of this research has been lost or ignored, but it deserves mention in order to stimulate further discussion and open doors to more investigation of the safety and effectiveness of magnesium.

The scientific research on magnesium that Rodale reported in his book highlighted the work of a brilliant French surgeon named Pierre Delbet. His interest in magnesium spread to many other doctors in France, who expanded his work. Rodale gives a long list of French physicians who over the years verified Dr. Delbet's findings and made new ones of their own. Delbet's magnesium research began while he was searching for a suitable antiseptic solution to apply to the wounds of soldiers injured in World War I and discovered that magnesium chloride had wonderful healing properties when applied externally.

IMMUNE SYSTEM

After judging magnesium chloride to be a very effective antiseptic solution, Dr. Delbet began testing oral forms of it on dogs and then with his patients, finding it to be a powerful immune system booster. In a paper presented to the French Academy of Medicine in September 1915, Delbet describes the effect on white blood cells of a solution of magnesium chloride injected into the veins of dogs. White blood cells from a blood sample taken before and after the injection were tested for their microbe-killing ability. Rodale reports that "five hundred white cells in the first sample destroyed 245 microbes. Five hundred white cells from the second destroyed 681. This increase in microbe-killing under the influence of magnesium chloride was 180 percent over the other solutions. More experiments were performed; in one there was an increase to 129 percent, in another, 333 percent."

POLIO

Fortunately, polio is not the scourge it once was. However, a follower of Dr. Delbet, Dr. Neveu, published a booklet titled *Therapeutic Treatment of Infectious Diseases by Magnesium Chloride: Poliomyelitis.* The book described fifteen cases of polio effectively treated with magnesium chloride. Neveu was so convinced of the effectiveness of magnesium chloride that he insisted that every home should have a solution of magnesium chloride on hand to treat the first signs of sore throat, especially when stiffness of the neck was involved. His formula was 20 grams of magnesium chloride powder to 1 liter of water.

SEIZURES

Rodale found evidence that seizures could be treated with magnesium. Dr. Lewis B. Barnett, head of the Hereford Clinic and Deaf Smith Research Foundation in Hereford, Texas, learned that magnesium is low in people with epilepsy. In the 1950s he presented evidence on thirty cases of childhood seizures that responded exceptionally well to high oral doses of magnesium. Barnett found that as his patients' blood magnesium reached normal levels, their seizure activity diminished. He also reported that the treatment was entirely harmless. As a result of his research, Barnett reported that the main cause for the 3 million clinical and 10–15 million subclinical cases of epilepsy identified at the time was a deficiency of magnesium.

CANCER

With one in two men and one in three women developing cancer in their lifetime, it's important to mention the relationship of this serious condition to magnesium deficiency. Dr. Mildred Seelig wrote a detailed paper on cancer and its interaction with minerals and vitamins with a focus on magnesium (available at www.mgwater.com/cancer.shtml). She noted a relationship between magnesium deficiency and cancer, which should have alerted the cancer establishment to do further research. J. I. Rodale wrote a chapter on cancer and magnesium in his 1963 publication with evidence from doctors in France of its importance.

Dr. Delbet felt that magnesium acts as a "brake" for cancer. He also observed that as the body grows older it grows more deficient in magnesium, and with this loss in magnesium there is a decrease in vitality, resistance, and cell regeneration.

PROSTATE

There appears to be no medical cure for swelling of the prostate (benign prostatic hypertrophy, or BPH) that leads to frequent nighttime urination. However, in 1930 Dr. Delbet and another doctor made two separate presentations to the Medical Academy of France showing that magnesium chloride could adequately treat this condition.

SENILITY AND AGING

It appears that the early French researchers were very aware of the problem caused by calcium precipitating into the tissues of the body. Dr. Delbet observed that with age, the body's tissues have three times more calcium than magnesium, and he concluded that magnesium deficiency plays a role in senility.

ALCOHOLISM

In his research, Delbet came to the conclusion that a major cause of alcoholism is magnesium deficiency. Unfortunately, there is little research being done on this association and even less on the clinical application of magnesium in the treatment of alcoholism in spite of the fact that medical researchers comment on alcoholism's association with magnesium deficiency.

MAGNESIUM AND BODY ODOR

There are no scientific studies about the effects of magnesium on body odor, but Rodale reported in his book that Delbet considered body odor to be due to an imbalance in the normal intestinal bacteria and that magnesium somehow restored that balance. Rodale later collected many anecdotal reports about the reduction of underarm odor, stool odor, and general body odor in people taking magnesium.

CHAPTER TWELVE

CHRONIC FATIGUE SYNDROME AND FIBROMYALGIA

THREE THINGS YOU NEED TO KNOW ABOUT MAGNESIUM, CHRONIC FATIGUE SYNDROME, AND FIBROMYALGIA

1. Magnesium deficiency is common in chronic fatigue syndrome and fibromyalgia sufferers.
2. Magnesium forms an important part of treatment for chronic fatigue syndrome and fibromyalgia.
3. Magnesium ameliorates the fatigue, muscle pain, and chemical sensitivity of chronic fatigue syndrome and fibromyalgia.

Over the past one hundred years, we have had a tremendous love affair with chemicals and electronics and a strange marriage with scientific methodology. It is safe to say that important advances in chemicals, pharmaceuticals, and science in general came out of the World War II effort and space research. The unseen potential risks to the public were presumably outweighed by the crisis of the time.

However, our sedentary lifestyle, consumption of synthetic foods, environmental chemicals, and polluted atmosphere have coincided with a greater frequency of chronic fatigue syndrome and fibromyalgia. On a parallel track, magnesium and other nutrients have become woefully depleted and, as we will see in Chapter 13, leave us unable to protect our bodies and brains from chemicals.

CHRONIC FATIGUE SYNDROME

Chronic fatigue syndrome (CFS) was formally recognized and defined as an illness by the Centers for Disease Control (CDC) in 1988. Before that time, and even since, many doctors considered the condition psychological. CFS goes by various names: Epstein-Barr, yuppie flu, and, in Britain, myalgic encephalomyelitis (which identifies the muscles and brain as sites of inflammation). Unfortunately, chronic fatigue syndrome is the name that has stuck in the United States, which makes it seem related to the generalized fatigue that anyone can suffer at one time or another. The name minimizes the global impact that this devastating disease can have on a person's life.

The symptoms of CFS are chronic headaches, swollen glands, periodic fevers and chills, muscle and joint aches and pains, muscle weakness, sore throat, and numbness and tingling of the extremities. The general feeling is one of incredible fatigue and inability to do even the simplest of tasks without becoming exhausted, inability to cope with any stress, and insomnia.

There are many theories about the cause of CFS, but one triggering factor could be a reactivation of an already present mononucleosis-like virus called Epstein-Barr virus. Upward of 90 percent of the population already has antibodies to Epstein-Barr virus, meaning the virus infected them at some point in their lives. In most people the infection came and went like a normal cold or flu. But for some, the first infection or the reactivation of the virus can be quite severe and leave them feeling fatigued, run-down, and never truly healthy again.

If CFS is some type of infection presenting itself in a new way, then the people it affects most severely seem to be more run-down and stressed than average. It appears that this infection becomes chronic because the immune system is not strong enough to fight it off or because sufferers come in contact with a chemical or pollutant that undermines their resistance and allows them to succumb to the illness. One of the ways the immune system is stressed is by the generalized depletion of minerals and vitamins that it needs to function properly.

CHRONIC FATIGUE SYNDROME DIAGNOSTIC CRITERIA

MAJOR CRITERIA
- New onset of fatigue, causing a 50 percent reduction in activity for at least six months
- Exclusion of other illnesses that can cause fatigue

MINOR CRITERIA
- Presence of eight of eleven symptoms, or six of eleven symptoms and two of the three signs

Symptoms
- Mild fever
- Recurrent sore throat
- Painful lymph nodes
- Muscle weakness
- Muscle pain
- Prolonged fatigue after exercise

- Recurrent headache
- Migratory joint pain
- Neurological or psychological complaints: sensitivity to bright light, forgetfulness, confusion, inability to concentrate, excessive irritability, depression
- Sleep disturbance
- Sudden onset of symptom complex

Signs

- Low-grade fever
- Sore throat without signs of pus
- Palpable or tender lymph nodes

Sheila fit the profile of chronic fatigue syndrome. After suffering mononucleosis during college, she has never felt quite the same. The mono seemed to weaken her immune system and her adrenal glands. Sheila worked as a teacher and was constantly exposed to germs, coming down with every cold and flu that passed through the school. Because she traveled a lot, she received numerous inoculations, which further weakened her. In her spare time she enjoyed furniture refinishing, which exposed her to tung oil, found in varnishes, paint strippers, and paint. Tung oil is made from euphorbia, a plant that produces phorbol esters, and has been proposed as a causative agent for chronic fatigue syndrome.[1]

After a trip to the Far East, Sheila became more and more fatigued and came down with a terrible month-long flu with a horribly achy head, muscles, and joints. Her doctor put her on one antibiotic after another, even though she had no bacterial infection. Her cough and chest pain finally cleared up, but she continued to have periodic fevers, a sore throat, and sore muscles. She couldn't exercise at all because she would end up in bed for days, and no matter how tired she was, she couldn't sleep. Sheila was depressed by this constant sickness. Sometimes she felt as if she were losing her mind: she couldn't concentrate, remember, or perform simple arithmetic. She couldn't teach and was so exhausted that she could do only the bare minimum to take care of herself.

Fortunately, Sheila's doctor was involved with a study at a local university looking into possible drug treatments for CFS. Sheila entered the blind study and did not know which treatment she was receiving. The three medications were an anti-inflammatory drug (ibuprofen), an antidepressant (amitriptyline), and magnesium glycinate. She had weekly visits with a nurse to assess her symptoms, twenty-four-hour urine collections, blood tests, and questionnaires. After two weeks her fatigue improved, as did her muscle weakness, twitching, poor concentration, and irritability.

At the end of the study, Sheila was told that her treatment had been 300 mg of elemental magnesium twice a day, that her magnesium had been very low at the beginning of the study, and that she could safely continue with the treatment if she wished. Sheila now had the energy to do more things to take care of herself: exercise, shop for the right foods, and prepare more meals from fresh foods. She knew she was on the road to recovery, thanks to magnesium. Several other studies confirm the efficacy of using magnesium for the treatment of chronic fatigue syndrome symptoms.[2, 3, 4, 5]

FIBROMYALGIA DIAGNOSTIC CRITERIA

MAJOR CRITERIA
- Generalized aches or stiffness of at least three anatomical sites for at least three months

- Six or more typical, reproducible tender points, called trigger points, in the muscles
- Exclusion of other disorders that can cause similar symptoms

MINOR CRITERIA
- Generalized fatigue
- Chronic headaches
- Sleep disturbances
- Neurological and psychological complaints
- Joint swelling
- Numbness or tingling sensation
- Irritable bowel syndrome
- Variation of symptoms in relation to activity, stress, and weather changes

FIBROMYALGIA

It wasn't until 1990 that the American College of Rheumatology established diagnostic criteria for fibromyalgia, thereby giving it official status as an illness. *Fibro* means "connective tissue" and refers to the thin tissue that wraps around muscles, and *myalgia* means "muscle pain." Also called fibrositis, fibromyalgia is a close cousin of CFS and shares many of its symptoms: incapacitating fatigue, muscle and joint pain, neuralgia, sleep disorders, anxiety, depression, cognitive confusion, and digestive problems. (CFS sufferers, in addition, have mild fever, swollen glands, and a sore throat, which distinguishes them from fibromyalgia patients.) Having a name, however, does not define the causes of the illness, and the American College of Rheumatology does not offer a curative treatment.

I believe fibromyalgia is the latest label for an accumulation of toxins and infections from both environment and lifestyle. Twenty-six doctors who present their cases in a book on chronic fatigue and fibromyalgia agree.[6]

Our exposure to toxins, chemicals, and prescription drugs begins at birth. Substances we think are safe can break down our immune systems and deplete our nutrient reserves. I and many other doctors believe they lead to CFS, fibromyalgia, and environmental illness in a growing list of sufferers.[7] Here's a chronology of ailments and the kinds of treatments any one of us may receive over the course of a lifetime. Each treatment can trigger the next event and further drug intervention. However, in my experience, a person with fibromyalgia can diminish his or her symptoms by 50 percent by taking the right amount of magnesium. In order to get sufficient magnesium into the tissues of the body that may mean taking IV magnesium, or more conveniently, applying magnesium oil or gel on the body. See Chapter 18 for detailed information.

POSSIBLE HEALTH CHRONOLOGY FOR CFS AND FIBROMYALGIA SUFFERERS

- Diaper rash, caused by *Candida albicans* (yeast), is mistakenly treated with cortisone creams, which encourage further growth of the yeast.
- Childhood ear infections can begin at birth as yeast infections picked up from the mother during delivery. Most ear infections are treated with antibiotics.
- Ear infections may become chronic and require multiple courses of antibiotics, leading to diarrhea and intestinal yeast infections.
- Anesthetics used in surgery to place tubes in the ears add another toxin.
- Colic can develop due to antibiotics.
- Inability to digest milk due to an irritated bowel leads to frequent changes of formula and further irritation.

- Gas and bloating can result from hard-to-digest soy formula.
- Eczema, aggravated by food sensitivity, is suppressed with cortisone creams.
- Allergies to foods, especially yeast, wheat, and dairy, can arise from poor digestion.
- Asthma, which may be environmental, is treated with medications including corticosteroid inhalers.
- Multiple colds and flus are mistreated with many courses of antibiotics.
- Annual flu vaccines contain mercury preservative.
- Cravings for sweets can be caused by yeast overgrowth and may cause or aggravate hyperactive behavior in children.
- Dental cavities lead to multiple mercury amalgam fillings. Toxic mercury vapor may be inhaled or absorbed, disrupting enzymes in the brain, kidneys, and liver.
- Allergic reactions are treated with allergy shots, antihistamines, and cortisone sprays.
- Many adolescents take long-term oral antibiotics for acne.
- Many teens and young adults develop mononucleosis, and up to 20 percent never feel quite as healthy again.
- Bladder infections are treated with antibiotics, which cause yeast infections.
- Birth control pills cause chronic vaginal yeast infections, which are mistreated with antibiotic creams.
- Pregnancy hormones encourage vaginal yeast infections.
- Chronic sleep deprivation is common in all parents of small children and is a major stress on the immune system.
- Irritable bowel syndrome can develop after a bout of

diarrhea (attributed to traveler's diarrhea or food poisoning) and is usually treated with antibiotics.

- Chronic sinus infections (97 percent are fungal, according to the Mayo Clinic) occur due to lowered immune system and are mistakenly treated with antibiotics.
- Hypothyroidism often occurs but remains undiagnosed and untreated.
- Hospitalization for infections or surgery usually warrants intravenous antibiotics and a host of other drugs.
- Major colds and flus can lead to bronchitis and pneumonia, which are treated with strong antibiotics.
- Chronic fatigue syndrome and fibromyalgia are treated with anti-inflammatories, sleeping pills, and antidepressants.
- Environmental allergies with extreme sensitivities to inhalants, especially perfumes, colognes, household products, pesticides, and molds, are treated with corticosteroid inhalers.
- Dysmenorrhea, irregular periods, infertility, and worsening premenstrual symptoms occur due to a buildup of toxins and lack of nutrients.
- Infertility is treated with an array of synthetic hormonal drugs.
- Depression, anxiety, panic attacks, and palpitations are treated with antidepressants and psychotherapy.
- Menopause is medicated with synthetic hormones.

Magnesium is depleted with every step of this scenario and results in a total body burden of drugs, toxins, and various stressors. The end result looks very much like chronic fatigue syndrome.

Let's look at the journey through life from the ground up to understand why we have become so nutrient-deficient and how this affects the immune system.

Plants grown on devitalized, overworked soil that has been poisoned by acid rain are poor in nutrients, including magnesium. The topic of magnesium-deficient soil is covered in Chapter 2. Synthetic foods created by modern processing and refining are devoid of natural vitamins, minerals, and fiber. They are "fortified" with useless synthetic vitamins and often no minerals except calcium or iron. Magnesium is the nutrient hardest hit by food processing.

The body is not able to adequately process junk food, with its dozens of chemical additives. It treats these chemical additives like foreign invaders and has to detoxify them in the liver. The intermediary metabolites are sometimes more toxic than the original, leaving the body hypersensitive and hyperimmune, sometimes turning on the body and creating autoimmune disease (such as multiple sclerosis or rheumatoid arthritis). Magnesium is depleted in the attempt to detoxify the body of these foreign chemicals.

There are thousands of medicinal drugs currently in use. Magnesium expert Dr. Mildred Seelig tells us that the side effects of many drugs may be associated with magnesium deficiency because magnesium becomes depleted while the body is trying to detoxify these drugs.

With the advent of antibiotics and the hope that they could cure all our infectious diseases, there is an overuse of these powerful drugs. When antibiotics kill bacteria, they cannot discriminate; they kill both good and bad bacteria. The good bacteria killed in the gastrointestinal tract are then replaced with yeast (*Candida albicans*).

The birth control pill, with its daily hormone surge, feeds yeast in the gut, as do sugar products. Yeast overgrowth results in episodes of alternating diarrhea and constipation. Magnesium is lost due to diarrhea and is drained by the constant demand to balance the pH of the body due to the acidity of soda pop and junk food.

The symptoms from yeast and its breakdown products are bodywide. Often these symptoms lead one to think that there are infections in the sinuses, throat, bladder, or vagina. A doctor will consequently prescribe more antibiotics for these symptoms, which merely perpetuates the problem. Overgrowth of yeast in the intestines can cause micropunctures in their lining, called *leaky gut*, thus allowing the absorption of incompletely digested food into the bloodstream. These undigested food particles are now foreign bodies, and the immune system reacts by forming antibodies to try to get rid of them. Food allergies and sensitivities result.

Allergies are created when inhaled chemicals and toxins irritate the mucous membranes of the nasal passages. They can trigger symptoms of asthma, which is made worse by magnesium deficiency.

Depression can be a direct result of accumulating chemicals in the body from drugs, synthetic food, and infections. When the brain is deficient in magnesium it is no longer protected from the onslaught of chemicals such as aspartame and MSG.

Because there are no medical tests to confirm that chemicals, drugs, and synthetic food are causing our symptoms, people who feel sick are often told that "everything is normal." This is frustrating and depressing, which makes sufferers feel even more unwell. The majority of chronically ill patients who come to my office or consult me by phone have seen between six and thirty doctors in one year for their complaints. Patients with fatigue or depression have usually been referred to a psychiatrist. Some patients have been prescribed thousands of dollars' worth of drugs annually to treat their multiple complaints, which usually have done no good and merely added to their toxin load.

The complex nature of CFS and fibromyalgia is formidable. Even though more doctors understand and accept the existence of CFS, the focus of CFS research seems to be on finding one cause. And the treatments offered are only symptomatic: rheumatologists and psychiatrists treat sleeplessness with sleeping pills; pain with antiinflammatory drugs, painkillers, and muscle relaxants; and anxiety and depression with anti-anxiety drugs and antidepressants. No attention is paid to diet or nutrient deficiencies. They ignore the possibility that there could be a nutrient imbalance, such as a magnesium deficiency, or coexisting conditions, such as a yeast infection, low thyroid, or allergies, that cause a complex of symptoms. They also tend to overlook possible toxicities, which allow common infections to appear more virulent as they take advantage of a weakened host. Yet magnesium deficiency is known to exacerbate all the symptoms of CFS and fibromyalgia, and increased magnesium intake has been effective in helping to restore health to many sufferers. Magnesium is also one of the best ways to strengthen the immune system and boost resistance against germs.

Exercise is often suggested for people suffering from fatigue, but even the mildest aerobic exercise is exhausting to people with CFS or fibromyalgia, who have no energy because their magnesium-driven energy system is bankrupt. Exercise also causes lactic acid buildup, which leads to more pain when it is not cleared by a particular enzyme that requires magnesium. Even the work of metabolizing pain medications depletes magnesium. This explains why chronic fatigue patients do not do well on most medications.

A buildup of lactic acid in the muscles causes pain and can be treated with 300 mg of elemental magnesium twice a day. If the joints accumulate toxicity, arthritis can occur; if the nerves are irritated by neurotoxins, they begin to lose their myelin sheath, and MS can result. In fact, autoimmune disease may also be the end stage of a buildup of toxicity along with a deficiency of nutrients, such as magnesium, that are designed to clear toxins from the body. According to some doctors, the definition of autoimmune disease as "disease against self" is not accurate; the disease process is, in fact, attacking a self altered by toxins and nutrient deficiencies.

Patients with fibromyalgia also have chronically low levels of serotonin, which greatly exaggerates their pain. As mentioned previously, magnesium is a necessary building block for both the production and uptake of serotonin by brain cells.

STRESS

Acute episodes of CFS and fibromyalgia are often brought on by exposure to stress, whether emotional or physical. The consequent increase in adrenaline and stress chemicals hastens magnesium loss and can be a factor in both these conditions. Low levels of magnesium intensify the secretion of the stress chemicals, thus increasing the risk of adverse effects of stress and creating another vicious circle.[8]

FATIGUE

The overproduction of adrenaline due to stress leads to magnesium deficiency and therefore puts a strain on the magnesium-dependent energy system of the body, causing energy depletion that leads to fatigue. Fatigue is often reduced with magnesium supplementation. In fact, a major breakthrough occurred in CFS research when low magnesium levels were discovered in most sufferers. Of the many enzyme systems that require magnesium, the most important ones are responsible for energy production and storage.

Magnesium and malic acid, an acid found in apples, are both crucial to the body's energy production and useful in the treatment of CFS and fibromyalgia. In the case of fibromyalgia, low magnesium keeps muscles in a state of spasm, so supplementation can aid in relieving this painful symptom. A study by Guy D. Abraham, M.D., showed positive results in the reversal of fibromyalgia with magnesium and malic acid supplementation. Fifteen patients with fibromyalgia who took magnesium (300–600 mg) and malic acid (1,200–2,400 mg) experienced improvement in their symptoms within the first forty-eight hours. Over an eight-week period of supplementation their degree of muscle tenderness and pain dropped from 19.6 points to 6.5 points, according to standardized medical scores.[9]

TREATMENT FOR CHRONIC FATIGUE AND FIBROMYALGIA

The treatment for CFS and fibromyalgia should address yeast overgrowth and IBS. Read *The Yeast Connection and Women's Health* (Crook and Dean, 2005) and *IBS for Dummies* (Dean and Wheeler, 2005). Diet and supplements should focus on building the immune system and the digestive system. Supplements touted for these conditions are many and varied but should be individualized with the help of a caring and knowledgeable practitioner. Oral magnesium supplements and magnesium oil or gel should form the cornerstone of therapy. Magnesium oil has the ability to increase the body's production of DHEA, a hormone that has beneficial effects on memory, stress, sleep, and depression, and naturally enhancing its effects will be very helpful for CFS and fibromyalgia. In my experience, using magnesium and treating yeast overgrowth can result in overall improvement of CFS and fibromyalgia of about 70–80 percent. Further improvement comes from treating low thyroid, estrogen dominance, and heavy metal toxicity.

CHAPTER THIRTEEN

ENVIRONMENTAL ILLNESS

THREE THINGS YOU NEED TO KNOW ABOUT MAGNESIUM AND ENVIRONMENTAL ILLNESS

1. Symptoms of chemical sensitivity can be completely or partially produced by magnesium deficiency.
2. Magnesium helps detoxify toxic chemicals.
3. Magnesium binds with and helps eliminate heavy metals from the body.

Dr. Sherry Rogers is a diplomate in family practice, allergy-asthma-immunology, and environmental medicine and a fellow of the American College of Nutrition. In private practice for more than thirty years, she treats very ill people from all over the world who have environmental toxicity and chemical sensitivity. The condition is called multiple chemical sensitivity (MCS) because a susceptible person usually has sensitivities to more than one chemical.

One of Dr. Rogers's basic maxims is that symptoms of chemical sensitivity can be wholly or in part produced by magnesium deficiency. She has tested enough people over the decades to know this to be a fact, and part of her success derives from implementing magnesium therapy for all her patients. Dr. Rogers notes that Dr. Frederica P. Perera, professor of environmental health sciences and director of the Columbia Center for Children's Environmental Health, has indicated that there is as much as a 500-fold difference in the ability of individuals to detoxify the same chemical. One of the key markers of this difference is each individual's magnesium level.

CFS and fibromyalgia are actually aspects of environmental illness. In Chapter 12 we saw how these conditions develop over time in a toxic environment. Now we will take a closer look at some environmentally sensitive people and the chemicals they encountered.

Natalie, sometimes in jest but more often in anger, would call what she experienced a "chemical warfare attack." It happened when she stepped out onto her driveway and was enveloped by a cloud of chemical spray from a lawn care truck treating her neighbor's yard. She could neither breathe nor speak. Her lungs were on fire, and her head felt as though it were exploding. She felt dizzy and shaky. She managed to stagger into the house, where she collapsed on the floor. Her husband found her a few minutes later and took her to the hospital, where they could do very little except give her oxygen and tell her to rest.

Natalie had been the picture of health—athletic, active, and happy. Now she was chronically fatigued. She became hypersensitive to every chemical she came in contact with. She couldn't even read; magazines and newspapers reeked of ink. Perfume samples that came in magazines were a nightmare. She had to find natural substitutes for cleaning products and cosmetics. Plants with moldy-smelling dirt had to go. She became allergic to wool. Her husband had to do all the cooking because she was sensitive to the gas fumes from their stove.

Her diet became increasingly limited, as she reacted to many foods. When she couldn't even use the telephone because holding the plastic receiver gave her hives, she became a prisoner in her own home with no contact with the outside world.

Elizabeth, Ted, and their children developed an array of symptoms after they used urea formaldehyde insulation in their home renovation. As soon as it was installed, they noticed an odor. The contractor said not to worry, it would be gone in a few days. The only thing that was gone in a few days was the contractor. They phoned and phoned, but he never returned their calls. By the end of the week the whole family had what appeared to be a bad cold, their eyes and noses streaming. The children developed skin rashes, and they all were irritable, headachy, and tired. When the "cold" didn't go away in ten days they went to the doctor, who saw their red, irritated skin and mucous membranes but no signs of infection, except for swollen neck glands. The doctor suggested they might be allergic to something. That clinched it; they knew it was the insulation. They didn't know what they could do about it. They tried toughing it out to see if the chemical would dissipate, but when the central heating came on the next month the problem actually got worse. They were beginning to be allergic to more and more things, and none of them felt well at all. Finally, they decided to rip out all the insulation, no matter what it cost.

Natalie, Elizabeth, Ted, and the children eventually got better. With much time, effort, and money and the help of sympathetic and knowledgeable health practitioners who understand the effects of the environment and the need to detoxify and nourish the body, they regained their health. The modalities they used were pure alkaline water, fresh air, organic foods, rotation diets, sauna therapy, vitamin and mineral supplements (especially 300 mg of elemental magnesium twice a day), homeopathy, acupuncture, and a positive attitude.

Some people with the above conditions are not as fortunate as Natalie, Elizabeth, and Ted, who at least knew what was harming them almost from the start. Those who gradually build up allergies and sensitivities to environmental toxins never know they're getting sick until they've developed asthma, eczema, or even cancer. What follows is an overview of our chemical environment and how its impact on our health can be lessened by neuroprotectants like magnesium.

In an important environmental study, toxic chemicals were found in nearly all foods tested by the FDA at levels consistent with negative health effects. They included persistent organic pollutants such as DDT and dioxin, which have been banned in the United States for decades but are still produced in other countries. Exposure to minuscule levels of these chemicals at crucial times in fetal and infant development can disrupt or damage human hormone, reproductive, neurological, and immune systems.[1]

In 2000 the Centers for Disease Control released the very first large-scale national survey of environmental toxins from human samples, and the results are startling. Blood and urine levels of twenty-seven chemicals tested in 5,000 Americans far exceeded safe levels. The EPA and CDC mostly rely on air, water, and soil samples to test for toxic levels of chemicals. Even then, only a few dozen of the more than 100,000 chemicals in everyday use are monitored for safety.[2] Hopefully this human study will reinforce a cutback in chemical pesticide use, as pledged by the U.S. Department of Agriculture (USDA) and the U.S. Environmental Protection Agency (EPA) in 1993. Chemical pesticide use, however, has increased from 900 million pounds in 1992 to 940 million pounds in 2000, while total cropland has decreased. And the riskiest chemical pesticides, such as organophosphates and carbamates, probable or possible carcinogens, still account for over 40 percent of the pesticides used in U.S. agriculture.[3]

The average American household generates fifteen pounds of household hazardous waste each year, according to the Texas Natural Resource Conservation Commission. "Our homes contain an average of three to eight gallons of hazardous materials in kitchens, bathrooms, garages and basements," the government agency reports. And what is the consequence of all these chemicals in our home environment? In a California study the number of people with sensitivities to one or more common chemicals is "surprisingly large," according to researchers. Just over 6 percent of the subjects reported having a diagnosis of multiple chemical sensitivity or environmental illness, and nearly 16 percent reported being allergic or unusually sensitive to everyday chemicals.[4]

In 1989, the World Health Organization took a strong stand regarding the origins of cancer when it stated that up to 80 percent of cancers are environmentally influenced. In 1985, the U.S. Environmental Protection Agency published a survey of human fat composition. It found that more than 99 percent of the population had measurable levels of the nine chemicals they tested for, including PCBs and DDT. In 2000, 100 percent of fat samples tested were positive for chemicals. Dr. Samuel Epstein, professor of occupational and environmental medicine at the University of Illinois Medical Center, Chicago, is an internationally recognized authority on the toxic and carcinogenic effects of environmental pollutants in air, water, and the workplace. His research was key to banning DDT and other problematic ingredients and contaminants in consumer products—food, cosmetics, and household products. In his keynote address to a Health Canada–sponsored cancer conference, he reported that we all now carry more than 500 different chemical compounds in our cells, none of which existed before 1920, and that "there is no safe dose for any of them."[5] With this information, activists have been demanding more use of safe alternatives to chemicals. But government and industry are still not listening.

Chemicals can destroy or paralyze different enzymes that protect us from external toxins. Thus, being exposed to chemicals prevents the body from protecting us from those very chemicals. Magnesium is active in more than 325 enzyme systems in the body, and when its enzymes are paralyzed, it is unable to do its essential work of energy production, detoxification, and brain and nerve protection.

METALS AND MAGNESIUM

Dr. Deborah Baker has researched the health effects of mercury for over a decade.[6] She acknowledges that mercury pervades our environment through industrial exposure, but the major source of elemental mercury in the general North American population is mercury vapor released from dental amalgams.[7, 8, 9, 10] These amalgams are, on average, 50 percent mercury, and they offgas, or vaporize, into your body's cells every time you chew, brush your teeth, or eat anything hot or acidic. There is a significant positive correlation between the number of amalgams in the mouth and the mercury content of human tissues, including the brain.[11]

Mercury drastically increases the excretion of magnesium and calcium from the kidneys, which may be the cause of the kidney damage seen in mercury poisoning.[12] Such mineral loss impairs cell production, the storage and utilization of energy, and cellular repair and replication. Sufficient magnesium supplementation can not only undo some of this damage but can prevent certain types of heavy metal toxicity.[13, 14]

Long-term fetal exposure during pregnancy to even low concentrations of mercury can lead to irreversible developmental disorders.[15] The concentration of magnesium in the placental and fetal tissues necessarily increases during pregnancy.[16] Unfortunately, the demand for magnesium usually exceeds its supply, and thus anything that further lowers magnesium levels, such as mercury, puts the pregnancy and child at risk.

Dr. Baker says that approximately 85 percent of her patients, as part of their mercury detoxification protocol, supplement with 300 mg to 500 mg daily of magnesium glycinate, in divided doses. Her patients frequently comment that their muscular pain improves while on magnesium.

Lead and cadmium have a cumulative toxic effect on the kidney and heart in particular. Magnesium appears to be a competitive inhibitor of these two polluting metals at different sites, particularly during combined intoxication.[17] A Yugoslavian research team found that increased intake of magnesium eliminates lead via the urine and may do the same with certain other heavy metals. Under experimental conditions, they found that magnesium increased excretion of cadmium via the urine.[18] Adequate magnesium levels can also help prevent the toxic effects of aluminum, which include breakdown of sugar stores and disruption in the production of ATP energy.[19] However, if magnesium levels are low, these heavy metals will stay in the body, binding to tissues in the kidney and heart and (in the case of aluminum especially) crossing the blood-brain barrier and destroying brain cells.

TREATMENT

The hallmark of a mineral-deficient person is often one who takes vitamins without minerals and feels worse or does well for a while but then deteriorates.[20] If you have a mineral deficiency, especially of magnesium, which is necessary for energy production, certain areas of the body may be overstimulated by vitamin supplements, while other areas can't respond. Therefore, if you suffer severe environmental illness, it is important to have a health care practitioner monitor supplement intake and to begin with magnesium as one of your first supplements.

The treatment for environmental illness is individualized. Since allopathic medicine does not recognize environmental disease, it has not established treatment protocols. According to environmental experts, magnesium is essential to build up the body's energy and fully utilize its detoxification systems. The source of environmental toxins, however, must be eliminated or avoided; otherwise it is like bailing out a sinking ship by hand. You first have to be aware of the chemicals in your environment, avoid them like the plague, and work diligently with the following therapies to clean out your body.

The lowly dry-cleaning chemicals, the mercury in dental fillings, and the cleaning products under the kitchen sink all build up in our bodies and cause chronic disease. Air purifying machines, water filters, organic food, organic supplements, and natural alternatives to chemicals provide the foundation of environmental health therapies.

DIET

The key in treating environmental illness is to eat organic, free-range, unprocessed, unadulterated foods. The pesticides added to the soil and the antibiotics used on poultry and beef sicken the animals and the people who eat them. The rash of diseases in cattle is likely related to the low quality of their feed, the tons of drugs they are given to fatten them up, and the gallons of chemicals sprayed on them to treat parasites. Unfortunately, even organic farms are subjected to acid rain, contaminated groundwater, and polluted air, which means that all of us should take an active role in detoxifying our bodies of suspected chemicals.

Drink six to eight glasses of pure water a day. Chemicals in our environment that are water-soluble are eliminated through the kidneys and colon, especially if you drink enough pure water. Use a water filter that has a pore size of less than 0.5 microns and guarantees the elimination of chemicals as well as parasites.

To eliminate fat-soluble chemicals such as pesticides and herbicides, which can become even more toxic when they are broken down by the liver, you need dry or far-infrared saunas. Fasting is not recommended to eliminate toxins. Fat-soluble chemicals are stored in fat cells, which keeps them out of circulation. When you try to fast or diet, your fat stores are broken down for energy, and out come the chemicals. The headache, nausea, light-headedness, and irritability are not just from lack of food but also from poisons flooding your bloodstream. While fasting, I've tasted and felt the numbing effect of dental anesthetics from decades before. If you are already feeling ill, fasting and dieting are going to be very unpleasant experiences.

DRY SAUNA

Numerous cultures use sweat lodges, steam baths, or saunas for cleansing and purification. Many health clubs and big apartment buildings have saunas and steam baths, and more and more people are building saunas in their own homes. Low-to-moderate-temperature saunas are one of the most important ways to detoxify from pesticide exposure. Head-to-toe perspiration through the skin, the largest organ of elimination, releases stored toxins and opens the pores. Fat that is close to the skin is heated, mobilized, and broken down, releasing toxins and breaking up cellulite. The heat increases metabolism, burns off calories, and gives the heart and circulation a workout. This is a boon if you don't have the energy to exercise. It is well known in medicine that a fever is the body's way of burning off an infection and stimulating the immune system. Fever therapy and sauna therapy are employed at alternative medicine healing centers to do just that. The controlled temperature in a sauna is excellent for relaxing muscular aches and pains and relieving sinus congestion. The only way I made it through my medical internship was by having regular saunas to reduce the daily stress.

FAR-INFRARED (FIR) SAUNAS

FIR saunas are inexpensive, convenient, and highly effective. Detox expert Dr. Sherry Rogers says that FIR is a proven and efficacious way of eliminating stored environmental toxins, and she thinks everyone should use one. There are one-person Sauna Domes that you lie under or more elaborate sauna boxes that seat several people. The far infrared provides a heat that increases the body temperature but the surrounding air is not overly heated. One advantage of the dome is that your head remains outside, which most people find more comfortable and less confining. Sweating begins within minutes of entering the dome and can be continued for thirty to sixty minutes. Besides the hundreds of toxins that can be removed through simple sweating, the heat of saunas creates a mild shock to the body, which researchers feel acts as a stimulus for the body's cells to become more efficient.

The outward signs are the production of sweat to help decrease the body temperature, but there is much more going on. Further research on sauna therapy is destined to make it an important medical therapy.

SUPPLEMENTS

If you have environmental illness, you feel as though you are sensitive or allergic to everything. When it comes to taking supplements, you may be unable to tolerate anything, but you might be deficient in everything. This does not necessarily mean that you are allergic to a particular supplement; rather, when you take it, your body responds by increasing some metabolic processes, which results in the body throwing off waste products that make you feel nauseated or headachy. That is why an organic diet, saunas, and exercise should be implemented before taking supplements.

The first supplement to add is magnesium and that can be in the form of a magnesium oil spray, which prevents rejection by the GI tract. Later, you can begin 100 mg of elemental magnesium (magnesium taurate or magnesium glycinate) once a day and add a second capsule after a week, a third in the third week, and a fourth a week later, in divided doses. Cut back if you have loose stools. "Green drinks" are the next food supplement to add. They are made from a variety of organic land and sea vegetables, and the better ones are flavored with stevia or nothing at all. Some green drinks are made with whey, hemp, or pea protein and make a good cleansing drink or meal replacement.

By now you should be feeling much better and able to add some more supplements under the guidance of a knowledgeable practitioner to help boost your immune system and provide necessary building blocks for health. Environmental illness does not require high-dose supplementation like other diseases. In fact, since most megavitamins and minerals are derived synthetically, it is a far better approach to use low-potency food-based supplements from organic sources.

===

CHAPTER FOURTEEN

ASTHMA

THREE THINGS YOU NEED TO KNOW
ABOUT MAGNESIUM AND ASTHMA

---

1. Research shows that many patients with asthma and other bronchial diseases have low magnesium.
2. Many drugs used in the treatment of asthma cause a loss of magnesium, only making symptoms worse.
3. Patients treated with simple magnesium supplementation report marked improvement in their symptoms.

As a child, Gerry had eczema. Every possible skin cream and lotion was tried, to no avail, but finally, after many years, the last patch disappeared on its own. It was followed almost immediately, however, by his first asthma attack. In his early thirties, Gerry was suffering attacks of wheezing and coughing when he exercised and when he was around cats, dogs, horses, dust, flowers, and chemical smells. Various inhalers helped initially, but after a year or two they would stop working. He wasn't satisfied with them, anyway; one gave him heart palpitations, and another contained steroids, which made him gain weight and retain fluid. Then one day a vitamin newsletter came in the mail. He almost threw it out, but a headline caught his attention: MAGNESIUM HALTS ASTHMA SPASMS.

Asthma is characterized by bronchial spasm, swelling of the mucous membranes of the lung, excessive mucus production, and an inability to fully empty the lungs of air. Asthma finds its easiest victims in children under ten and is twice as common in boys and men, although it affects about 3 percent of the general population. Tabulating all the triggers of an asthma attack is a daunting task; there seems to be a variety of stimuli, including lung infection, exercise, emotional upset, food sensitivities, inhalation of cold air or irritating aromatic substances (smoke, gas fumes, paint fumes, chemical fumes), and reactions to specific allergens, such as pollens.

Bronchial spasms occur in both extrinsic asthma (an allergic reaction to external substances such as mold, dust, animal hair, pollens, and chemicals) and intrinsic asthma (from exercise, infection, and emotional upset). The allergic triggers, called allergens, initiate the release of histamines in your body, which try to eliminate the allergens by stimulating lots of mucus to mop up the allergens and push them out through sneezing, coughing, and watery eyes. One of the side effects of too much histamine is tightening of the bronchial tubes, which go into spasm. Such spasms can initiate episodic wheezing, coughing, and shortness of breath, which quickly lead to rapid breathing, difficulty exhaling, anxiety, and dehydration. The anxiety of an asthma attack can create a gripping fear that tenses up the whole body and is hard to shake off.

Gerry really identified with what he read about asthma and magnesium in the newsletter. He realized that his whole body was tense. He decided to try some magnesium supplements under his doctor's supervision, and with them he was able to greatly decrease his medications.

Magnesium is an excellent treatment for asthma because it is a bronchodilator and an antihistamine, naturally reducing histamine levels in the body. It has a calming effect on the muscles of the bronchial tubes and the whole body. Certainly, drug therapy for asthma can often be lifesaving; drugs, however, are not curative. You have to eliminate the underlying cause of asthma and replace magnesium to fully treat this condition. Without magnesium, asthma can become chronic, especially if the various triggers are not eliminated; even the fear of an attack can magnify the emotional component. Conventional allergy shots have been used for decades to try to trick the body into accepting irritating allergens but often do not work, especially when the condition is due to a nutrient deficiency.

According to Dr. Mildred Seelig, the drug treatment of asthma consists of magnesium-wasters such as beta-blockers, corticosteroids, and Ventolin (albuterol). The side effects of these drugs include severe magnesium deficiency, which can result in arrhythmia and sudden death.[1] Taking theophylline (aminophylline) can cause loss of magnesium and suppression of vitamin B_6 activity, which is necessary for magnesium function. Prednisone wastes magnesium, causes sodium retention and fluid retention, suppresses vitamin D, and promotes increased urinary excretion of zinc, vitamin K, and vitamin C.[2]

Childhood asthma can be life-threatening, but safe methods of treating this condition are available and can be used along with medications. In a European study, a group of children who had deteriorated in spite of conventional drug therapy were given magnesium sulfate intravenously. Comparing the magnesium group with the placebo group, the magnesium group had lower clinical asthma scores and a significantly greater improvement in lung function over a ninety-minute period. No significant side effects were observed.[3]

Dr. Lydia Ciarallo in the Department of Pediatrics, Brown University School of Medicine, treated thirty-one asthma patients ages six to eighteen who were deteriorating on conventional treatments. One group was given magnesium sulfate and another group was given saline solution, both intravenously. At fifty minutes the magnesium group had a significantly greater percentage of improvement in lung function, and more magnesium patients than placebo patients were discharged from the emergency department and did not need hospitalization.[4]

Another study showed a correlation between intracellular magnesium levels and airway spasm. The investigators found that patients who had low cellular magnesium levels had increased bronchial spasm. This finding confirmed not only that magnesium was useful in the treatment of asthma by dilating the bronchial tubes but that lack of magnesium was probably a cause of this condition.[5]

A team of researchers identified magnesium deficiency as surprisingly common, finding it in 65 percent of an intensive-care population of asthmatics and in 11 percent of an outpatient asthma population. They supported the use of magnesium to help prevent asthma attacks. Magnesium has several antiasthmatic actions. As a calcium antagonist, it relaxes airways and smooth muscles and dilates the lungs. It also reduces airway inflammation, inhibits chemicals that cause spasm, and increases anti-inflammatory substances such as nitric oxide.[6]

The same study established that a lower dietary magnesium intake was associated with impaired lung function, bronchial hyperreactivity, and an increased risk of wheezing. The study included 2,633 randomly selected adults ages eighteen to seventy. Dietary magnesium intake was calculated by a food frequency questionnaire, and lung function and allergic tendency were evaluated. The investigators concluded that low magnesium intake may be involved in the development of both asthma and chronic obstructive airway disease.

DIET

Avoid sugar and white flour products. Limit red meat and dairy, which contain substances that increase inflammation in the body. Increase yellow vegetables and green leafy vegetables, which contain substances that inhibit inflammation. Increase intake of fish oils, seed and nut oils, cold-water fish (herring, sardines, salmon), flaxseed oil, and walnuts to reduce inflammation. Eat grapes; grape skins contain quercetin, which prevents histamine release and inhibits inflammatory products.

Try a liquid diet: use a whey, hemp, or pea protein powder, a green drink, and/or fresh, organic juices plus fiber for three days, followed by a vegetarian diet for four days.

Get out of the rut of eating the same foods every day; avoid your top three favorite foods to eliminate possible food allergies (people often crave foods they are sensitive to). Eggs, shellfish, and peanuts usually cause immediate sensitivity reactions; milk, chocolate, wheat, citrus, and food colorings cause delayed food reactions. Carefully check labels in the grocery store and speak up in restaurants to avoid even small amounts of potential allergic triggers such as MSG, aspartame, and sulfites.

Avoid aspirin and nonsteroidal anti-inflammatories (e.g., ibuprofen), which can cause allergic reactions.

Clean out environmental allergens: Find other homes for cats and dogs. Avoid wall-to-wall carpeting, wall hangings, and feather pillows. Frequently replace or clean air filters for heating and cooling systems. Obtain environmentally sound cleaning products. Use a vacuum cleaner specifically for allergies. Research HEPA air cleaners for your home. Since yeast overgrowth may be related to asthma, read *The Yeast Connection and Women's Health* (Crook and Dean, 2005) to understand the association.

SUPPLEMENTS FOR ASTHMA

Magnesium citrate: 300 mg twice a day
Vitamin B_6: 50 mg twice a day
Pantothenic acid: 500 mg daily
Vitamin C: 1–2 g daily
Vitamin E as mixed tocopherols: 400 IU daily
Quercetin (a bioflavonoid): 500 mg three times a day
Selenium: 250 mcg a day
Flaxseed oil: 1–2 tbsp daily
Hydrochloric acid: 5 grains, one tablet per day at the end of a
    meal, increasing to one with each meal
Probiotics: 2–10 billion living organisms per capsule, one in
    the morning and one in the evening before bed

===

CHAPTER FIFTEEN

HEALTH AND LONGEVITY

THREE THINGS YOU NEED TO KNOW
ABOUT MAGNESIUM AND AGING

1. Magnesium is deficient in people who have Alzheimer's disease or Parkinson's disease.
2. Aging itself is a risk factor for magnesium deficiency; as we get older we become more deficient in magnesium and therefore require more in our diet and in supplement form.
3. Magnesium oil applied to the skin stimulates production of DHEA, the antiaging hormone.

Three hundred years ago, people didn't live as long as we do today. They lived in such unsanitary conditions that simple scrapes and cuts became mortal wounds. Bathing was looked upon with suspicion. Tuberculosis, fostered by extremely close quarters, little sun exposure, dampness, and lack of fresh vegetables, was highly contagious and struck down many in their prime. Indoor fires without adequate ventilation caused chronic bronchitis and emphysema, if the people even lived long enough to develop these conditions.

When we implemented universal sanitation, the infectious diseases began to recede. The land was still fertile, and plants soaked up vital nutrients. Farm animals ate the plants, and humans absorbed the nutrients from eating fresh meat and fresh produce. The industrial revolution, however, harmed our health in a new way, with factories belching smoke and chemical poisons. Industrial farming techniques began poisoning the soil with pesticides, herbicides, and nitrogen fertilizers. The soil became lifeless.

We may think we are better off in this century with our drugs and medical technology, but as we've seen, these can also become toxic and undermine our health, especially in a polluted environment where our basic nutrition is impaired. Popping antiaging pills and megavitamins, however, does *not* add years to your life. An excellent diet that provides optimal nutrients, exercise, and an outgoing, optimistic attitude are the true keys to longevity.

Aging in industrialized societies is associated with an increasing prevalence of hypertension, heart disease, reduced insulin sensitivity, and adult-onset diabetes. Aging in general is associated with altered calcium and magnesium ion levels, indistinguishable from those observed in hypertension and diabetes.[1] As noted in the introduction to Part Three, French magnesium researcher Dr. Pierre Delbet, who practiced in the early 1900s, was convinced that the aging body's tissues have three times more calcium than magnesium. He knew that calcium precipitates out into tissues that have a deficiency of magnesium. He observed the toxicity of excess calcium in the testicles, brain, and other tissues and concluded almost a century ago that magnesium deficiency plays a role in senility. In Chapter 8 we talked about insulin resistance and its role in exacerbating hypertension, heart disease, and diabetes mellitus.

Insulin-resistant states, as well as what is often thought of as "normal" aging, are characterized by the accumulation of calcium and depletion of magnesium in the cells. With this in mind, clinical researchers in this century are finally suggesting that it is the disturbance of calcium and magnesium ions that might be the missing link responsible for the frequent clinical coexistence of hypertension, atherosclerosis, and metabolic disorders in aging.[2]

As is evident from animal experiments and epidemiological studies, magnesium deficiency may increase our susceptibility to cardiovascular disease as well as accelerate aging.[3] In a study of nursing home residents, low magnesium levels were significantly associated with two conditions that plague the elderly, calf cramps and diabetes mellitus.[4] Centenarians (individuals reaching a hundred years of age) have higher total body magnesium and lower calcium levels than most elderly people.[5]

> "Smart drugs" such as piracetam, oxiracetam, pramiracetam, and aniracetam are thought to enhance learning, facilitate the flow of information between the two hemispheres of the brain, help the brain resist physical and chemical injuries, and be relatively free of side effects. Magnesium fits all the criteria for "smart drugs," but it is much less costly and has no side effects.

FREE RADICALS, ANTIOXIDANTS, AND AGING

A free radical is an unstable molecule that is the product of normal body metabolism. It is formed when molecules within our own body's cells react with oxygen. It has an unpaired electron that tries to steal a stabilizing electron from another molecule and as a consequence can produce harmful effects. External sources of free radicals include chemicals (pesticides, industrial pollution, auto exhaust, cigarette smoke), heavy metals (dental amalgam, lead, cadmium), most infections (viruses, bacteria, parasites), X-rays, alcohol, allergens, stress, and even excessive exercise.

Antioxidants are vitamins and minerals such as magnesium, selenium, vitamin C, and vitamin E that turn off free radicals. The greater the amount of other antioxidants in the body, the more magnesium is spared from acting as an antioxidant and is free to perform its many other functions. So taking supplemental antioxidants protects the level of magnesium in the body; this prevents elevation of calcium, which can lead to vascular muscle spasm.[6] If there are not enough antioxidants available, overabundant free radicals begin to damage and destroy normal, healthy cells. Free radicals are necessary and normal products of metabolism, but uncontrolled free radical production plays a major role in the development of degenerative disease, since free radicals can damage any body structure: proteins, enzymes, fats, even DNA. Free radicals are implicated in more than sixty different health conditions, including heart disease, autoimmune disease, and cancer.

According to current research, low magnesium levels not only magnify free radical damage but can hasten the production of free radicals.[7] One study utilizing cultures of skin cells found that low magnesium doubled the levels of free radicals.[8] In addition, cells grown without magnesium were twice as susceptible to free radical damage as were cells grown in normal amounts of magnesium. Another study showed that red blood cells from hamsters fed low-magnesium diets were deficient in magnesium and consequently more susceptible to free radical damage. It appears that low magnesium damages the vital fatty layer in the cell membrane, making it more susceptible to destruction and allowing leakage through the membrane. This particular finding, which implicates magnesium deficiency as one of the causes of leaky cell membranes, is extremely important because disruption of this type can be fatal to cells and cause widespread problems that ultimately manifest in the list of conditions and symptoms of magnesium deficiency on pages 17–20.

A number of reports have identified pesticides as a cause of Parkinson's disease (which affects over a million Americans), with in-home exposure to insecticides carrying the highest risk.[9] Glutathione is a naturally occurring antioxidant made in all the cells of the body, including neurons, which acts to detoxify the body of certain chemicals. Cells grown in magnesium-deficient conditions, however, have lower glutathione levels. Adding free radicals to a low-magnesium cell culture causes the level of glutathione to fall rapidly as it is used up, making the cells much more susceptible to free radical damage. Neurosurgeon Dr. Russell Blaylock tells us that a fall in cellular glutathione within part of the brain called the substantia nigra appears to be one of the earliest findings in Parkinson's disease.[10]

MEMORY

It's much easier to view the tangible and structural benefits of magnesium—the bones, proteins, and even the energy it produces—but much more difficult to contemplate its effects on the brain. Research at MIT, however, produced a study in 2004 that elevates magnesium to the position of memory enhancer.

It appears that particular brain receptors important for learning and memory depend on magnesium for their regulation. The researchers describe magnesium as absolutely necessary in the cerebrospinal fluid in order to keep these learning and memory receptors active. The term they use for this activity, interactivity, and changeability is *plasticity*.

Plasticity decreases with age, and it's the loss of plasticity in the brain region responsible for storing short-term memories that causes forgetfulness in the elderly. Magnesium, they found, is instrumental in opening the receptor to important information, yet at the same time being able to ignore background noise. The researchers were quite struck by their findings and concluded, "As predicted by our theory, increasing the concentration of magnesium and reducing the background level of noise led to the largest increases of plasticity ever reported in scientific literature."[11]

ALZHEIMER'S

In North America, approximately 10 percent of the population over sixty-five and 50 percent over eighty-five suffer from Alzheimer's. It is associated with severe memory loss, impaired cognitive function, and inability to carry out activities of daily life. Alzheimer's disease should be diagnosed only when all the other identifiable brain conditions are ruled out (e.g., brain tumor, alcoholism, vitamin B_{12} deficiency, mercury amalgam poisoning, depression, hypothyroidism, Parkinson's, stroke, excessive prescription drug use, malnutrition, and dehydration). In truth, it is only at autopsy that a definitive diagnosis can be made, as the brain will show the identifying characteristics of Alzheimer's: plaques and tangles in the nerve fibers, particularly in the cerebral cortex and hippocampal area. Dr. Abram Hoffer, the founder of orthomolecular medicine along with Linus Pauling, cautions that almost half the cases of what is assumed to be Alzheimer's may in fact be dementias caused by such treatable conditions as simple dehydration, prescription drug intoxication, severe cerebral allergies to foods or chemicals, or chronic nutrient deficiencies. Drugs that worsen Alzeimer's include chlorpromazine, anti-histamines, barbiturates, psychotropic drugs, and diuretics.

Chemicals and toxic metals are associated with Alzheimer's disease, especially mercury and aluminum. The Alzheimer's-mercury connection has been made by Dr. Boyd Haley, a professor of chemistry and chair of that department at the University of Kentucky. Dr. Haley proved that the tangles and plaques in the Alzheimer's brain were identical to those produced by mercury poisoning. Mercury can be absorbed into the brain from dental amalgams, be acquired by taking flu shots (which are preserved with mercury), or come from habitually eating fish contaminated with mercury. Magnesium, when it is available in the body, will help detoxify heavy metals, even ones as poisoinous as mercury.

Many Americans are exposed to aluminum through aluminum pots, aluminum cans, aluminum-containing antacids and antiperspirants, aluminum foil, and tap water that may be high in aluminum.[12, 13] Considerable research has proven that brain neurons affected in Alzheimer's disease have significantly higher levels of aluminum than normal neurons. Alzheimer's patients also have consistently low magnesium levels within the hippocampus, the area of the brain most damaged by Alzheimer's. Aluminum is able to replace magnesium in certain enzyme systems in the body, mimicking its function but causing harm. Aluminum can also replace magnesium in the brain, which leaves calcium channels in the brain nerve cells wide open, allowing calcium to flood in, causing cell death.[14]

William Grant, an atmospheric scientist, had a personal interest in Alzheimer's because of a strong family history. Grant already knew that people with Alzheimer's typically have elevated concentrations of aluminum in their brains. He put that bit of information together with the fact that acid rain makes aluminum more abundant in trees and seems to make trees age prematurely. Grant theorized that the diets of Alzheimer's patients might be very acidic, leaching calcium and magnesium from the body. He found that people with Alzheimer's have elevated amounts of aluminum, iron, and zinc and have reduced amounts of alkali metals such as magnesium, calcium, and potassium, which neutralize the acidity in the diet. A typical Western diet—high in protein, fat, and sugar—is acid-forming and may be an additional factor in creating aluminum overload in Alzheimer's.

PARKINSON'S DISEASE

Similarly, aluminum can be a contributing factor in the central nervous system degeneration that occurs with Parkinson's disease. In one autopsy study, calcium and aluminum were elevated in the brains of victims of Parkinson's disease as compared to people with normal brains.[15]

Enzymes function in the body only when they have access to the proper cofactors, which are mostly vitamins and minerals, especially magnesium, selenium, vitamin C, vitamin B_6, and vitamin E. Heavy metals such as cadmium, aluminum, and lead attach themselves to certain enzymes, kicking out minerals such as magnesium, and either prevent the normal enzyme activity or create abnormal activity leading to cell destruction.

Research indicates that ample magnesium will protect brain cells from the damaging effects of aluminum, beryllium, cadmium, lead, mercury, and nickel. We also know that low levels of brain magnesium contribute to the deposition of heavy metals in the brain that heralds Parkinson's and Alzheimer's. It appears that the metals compete with magnesium for entry into the brain cells. If magnesium is low, metals gain access much more readily.

There is also competition in the small intestine for absorption of minerals. If there is enough magnesium, aluminum won't be absorbed. When monkeys are fed diets low in calcium and magnesium but high in aluminum, for instance, they become apathetic and begin to lose weight. When their spinal cords are examined under the microscope, they show swelling of the anterior motor cells (movement centers), plus accumulation of calcium and aluminum in these cells.[16] If you eat from aluminum pots, use aluminum-containing antiperspirants, wrap your food in aluminum foil, and drink tap water with high aluminum content, the levels could overwhelm the magnesium in your gut, and aluminum will be absorbed instead. This has consequences for the amount of magnesium in your brain and may allow the buildup of aluminum associated with Alzheimer's and Parkinson's disease.

Dr. Blaylock reports that when scientists study the soil of regions that have a high incidence of neurological diseases, they find high levels of aluminum and low levels of magnesium and calcium. The neurons from victims of the disease also show high levels of aluminum and low levels of magnesium. On the island of Guam the areas with the lowest levels of calcium and magnesium in the soil are also the areas of highest incidence for all neurological diseases. Magnesium plays a vital role in protecting neurons from the lethal effects of aluminum.[17]

MAGNESIUM-DEFICIENCY DEMENTIA

Dementia may also be caused by magnesium depletion alone.[18] Several studies show that severe neurological syndromes can result when conditions cause extremely low levels of brain magnesium, such as with the chronic use of diuretics, which millions of people take to control high blood pressure. These neurological conditions can present as seizures, delirium, coma, or psychosis, which are quickly reversed by administering large doses of intravenous magnesium.

The body's ability to absorb magnesium declines with age, so at particular risk are elderly people who do not eat an adequate diet and who use drugs that deplete the body's magnesium. (Studies show that senior citizens take on average six to eight medications regularly.) Add to that the effects of antacids, which many elderly people take to cover up symptoms caused by a bad diet. Antacids suppress normal stomach acid and can lead to incompletely digested food, which causes gas, bloating, and constipation. (As previously noted, another hidden danger is the use of aluminum in most antacids.)

Excessive amounts of aspartame and MSG (glutamate) in the diet of elderly people may also cause symptoms of dementia due to their direct effect, which is also magnified in magnesium deficiency.

AGING

Dr. Jean Durlach, a preeminent magnesium expert in France, sums up the current research on magnesium and aging.[19]

1. Chronic marginal magnesium deficiency reduces life span in rats.
2. Magnesium deficiency accelerates aging through its various effects on the neuromuscular, cardiovascular, and endocrine apparatus; kidneys and bones; and immune, antistress, and antioxidant systems.
3. In developed countries, magnesium intake is marginal throughout the entire population regardless of age: around 4 mg/kg/day instead of the 6 mg/kg/day recommended to maintain satisfactory balance. However, diseases, handicaps, and physical or

psychological impairments expose elderly individuals to more severe nutritional deficiencies.

4. Around the age of seventy, magnesium absorption is two-thirds of what it is at age thirty.

5. Various mechanisms of deficiency include intestinal malabsorption; reduced bone uptake and mobilization (osteoporosis); increased urinary losses; chronic stress; insulin resistance leading to diabetes with severe magnesium loss in the urine; lack of response to adrenal stimulation; loss caused by medication, especially diuretics; alcohol addiction; and cigarette smoking.

6. Magnesium deficiency symptoms in the elderly include central nervous system symptoms that seem largely "neurotic": anxiety, excessive emotionality, fatigue, headaches, insomnia, light-headedness, dizziness, nervous fits, sensation of a lump in the throat, and impaired breathing. Peripheral nervous system signs are common: pins and needles of the extremities, cramps, muscle pains. Functional disorders include chest pain, shortness of breath, chest pressure, palpitations, extra systoles (occasional heart thumps from an isolated extra beat), abnormal heart rhythm, and Raynaud's syndrome. Autonomic nervous system disturbances involve both the sympathetic and parasympathetic nervous systems, causing hypotension on rising quickly or borderline hypertension. In elderly patients, excessive emotionality, tremor, weakness, sleep disorders, amnesia, and cognitive disturbances are particularly important aspects of magnesium deficiency.

7. A trial of oral magnesium supplementation is the best diagnostic tool for establishing the importance of magnesium.

MAGNESIUM OIL AND DHEA

Dr. Norman Shealy found while resesarching magnesium oil that magnesium applied to the skin on a regular basis naturally enhances the level of a vitally important hormone, DHEA. DHEA is normally produced in the adrenal glands, but production slows down as we age. Apparently as magnesium is absorbed through the skin and the underlying fatty tissues of the body it sets off many chain reactions, one of which ends in the production of DHEA.

Increasing DHEA levels by taking supplements of the hormone is recommended by some antiaging specialists, but others caution about side effects. To increase it naturally by improving your magnesium balance may be a safe way to turn back the clock.

TREATMENT BEYOND MAGNESIUM

MANAGEMENT OF ALUMINUM TOXICITY AND ALZHEIMER'S

Use only filtered water, and ensure that the filter guarantees removal of aluminum; drink eight glasses per day. Check labels and avoid antacids containing aluminum. Use natural antiperspirants. Avoid cooking in aluminum pots or drinking fruit juice or soft drinks from aluminum containers. Get checked for thyroid disease and treat appropriately. Check for heavy metal toxicity (aluminum, mercury, copper, lead, and iron) through urine testing or hair analysis. Pursue either oral or intravenous chelation to remove your heavy-metal burden.

ALTERNATIVE THERAPIES FOR ALZHEIMER'S

Avoid mercury fillings or have them replaced; if you decide to have your mercury amalgams removed, find a practitioner who has been trained in their safe removal, as improper removal can result in more mercury being released into the tissues (see the Resources list). Clean out all the chemicals in your home and immediate environment. Eat organic food. Exercise and take regular saunas.

DIET FOR LONGEVITY

Avoid all junk food and salty, fried, and fatty foods. Stay away from meat, alcohol, coffee, caffeine, and sugar. Check for food sensitivities, particularly wheat and dairy. Therapeutic foods include cilantro, onion, seaweeds, and ginger, which help bind and excrete heavy metals.

SUPPLEMENTS FOR LONGEVITY

Magnesium citrate: 300 mg two or three times per day

Magnesium oil applied to the skin, 10–20 sprays per day; dilute by half with distilled water if the oil stings (each spray of undiluted oil carries about 20 mg of magnesium). Magnesium gel has less tendency to sting.

Calcium citrate: 500 mg daily

Vitamin E as mixed tocopherols: 400 IU daily

Vitamin C: 1,000 mg twice per day

B complex: 50 mg twice per day

Vitamin B_{12}: 1,000 mcg intramuscularly weekly

Vitamin D: 1,000 IU or 20 minutes of sun exposure daily.

Lecithin granules: 2 tbsp per day

Flaxseed oil: 1–2 tbsp per day

Fish oil (halibut liver oil or cod liver oil): 1 tsp per day

Ginkgo biloba and gotu kola are two herbs that can improve cerebral circulation.

PART FOUR

TESTING AND SUPPLEMENTS

CHAPTER SIXTEEN

MAGNESIUM REQUIREMENTS AND TESTING

It's confusing enough trying to determine your individual needs for magnesium without having to wade through the alphabet soup of guidelines set by government agencies, including the DRI, RDA, RDI, AI, UL, and EAR. In 1997, the Food and Nutrition Board of the National Academy of Sciences created the Dietary Reference Intakes (DRIs), which added more guidelines to the Recommended Dietary Allowances (RDAs) that were the standard from 1941 to 1989. Statistical analysis of diets for certain nutrients is necessary for the planning of menus to meet the nutrient needs of different age groups of people. They are also used to evaluate food consumption patterns and to create guidelines for nutrition labeling, all with an eye to preventing nutrient deficient diseases. This is an important point to remember: the RDA nutrient intake guidelines did not recommend levels for optimal health and vitality but told you how much vitamin C to take, for example, so you won't get scurvy, or vitamin B_1, so you won't get pellagra.

The DRIs are now made up of four different reference values: the Estimated Average Requirement (EAR), the Recommended Dietary Allowance (RDA), the Adequate Intake (AI), and the Tolerable Upper Intake Level (UL). The UL is most important because it focuses on higher intake levels than the RDA to reduce the risk of chronic diseases such as osteoporosis, cancer, and cardiovascular disease.

Implementation of the DRIs was done in stages from 1997 to 2005. Focusing on the prevention of osteoporosis, the first report, published in 1997, was the *Dietary Reference Intakes for Calcium, Phosphorus, Magnesium, Vitamin D and Fluoride*. Four additional reports have covered folate and other B vitamins; dietary antioxidants (vitamins C and E, selenium, and the carotenoids); the micronutrients (vitamins A and K, and trace elements such as iron, iodine, etc.); macronutrients such as dietary fat and fatty acids, protein and amino acids, carbohydrates, sugars, and dietary fiber, as well as energy intake and expenditure; electrolytes and water; bioactive compounds such as phytoestrogens and phytochemicals; and the role of alcohol in health and disease.

While the DRIs are used mainly by academic research scientists and nutritionists and are not a household word, doctors who focus on nutrition, such as myself, appreciate having the information in these reports. The confusing part in the magnesium report is that two different values are given for dietary magnesium and for supplemental magnesium. There is no total requirement and no acknowledgment that the level of magnesium in the average diet is less than half the RDA.

In 1997, the RDA of magnesium was raised 15 percent, from 350 mg/day to 420 for men and from 280 mg/day to 320 for women. However, the same 1997 report on the safe upper limit of dietary magnesium for adults states that "because magnesium has not been shown to produce any toxic effects when ingested as a naturally occurring substance in foods, a UL cannot be established for dietary magnesium at this time." The report also noted that "no specific toxicity data exist on which to establish a UL [for dietary magnesium] for infants, toddlers, and children." In determining the dietary magnesium UL for pregnant and breast-feeding women, it concluded that "studies involving intravenous administration of comparatively large doses of magnesium used in the treatment of preterm labor, pregnancy-induced hypertension, or other clinical conditions were not considered applicable for the derivation of ULs."

Looking at supplemental magnesium, the committee set what some consider to be a very low UL for pregnant and breast-feeding women, despite their high magnesium needs. Even though the report states that "no evidence suggests increased susceptibility to adverse effects of supplemental magnesium during pregnancy and lactation," they set the UL for this group at 350 mg (14.6 mmol)/day. This is the same UL for supplemental magnesium in adults who are not pregnant or lactating.

The report does concede that supplements above the UL may be necessary. "Individuals with impaired renal function are at greater risk of magnesium toxicity. However . . . magnesium levels obtained from food are insufficient to cause adverse reactions even in these individuals. Patients with certain clinical conditions (for example, neonatal tetany, hyperuricemia, hyperlipidemia, lithium toxicity, hyperthyroidism, pancreatitis, hepatitis, phlebitis, coronary artery disease, arrhythmia, and digitalis intoxication . . .) may benefit from the prescribed use of magnesium in quantities exceeding the UL in the clinical setting."

MAGNESIUM REQUIREMENTS

As noted, the Recommended Daily Allowance (RDA) for nutrients is set at the minimum level to stave off deficiency symptoms, not at the optimum that ensures good health. But even with the RDA set so low, most Americans are still deficient in magnesium, with men obtaining only about 80 percent of the recommended daily allowance (RDA) and women averaging only 70 percent.

The following table shows the Recommended Daily Allowances (RDAs) for magnesium in children and adults.

Children 1 to 3 years: 80 mg
Children 4 to 8 years: 130 mg
Children 9 to 13 years: 240 mg

Life Stage	Men	Women	Pregnancy	Lactation
Age 14–18	410 mg	360 mg	400mg	360 mg
Age 19–30	400 mg	310 mg	350 mg	310 mg
Age 31+	420 mg	320 mg	360 mg	320 mg

The RDA for magnesium is also expressed in mg/kg and is roughly 6 mg per kg (2.2 lb) of body weight. This standard helps to determine the magnesium requirements for someone who is overweight; a fifty-year-old who weighs 300 lbs needs more magnesium than a fifty-year-old who is 100 lbs.

Many magnesium experts feel that the RDA should be increased. Twenty years of research shows that under ideal conditions approximately 300 mg of magnesium is required merely to offset the daily losses. If you are under mild to moderate stress caused by a physical or psychological disease, physical injury, athletic exertion, or emotional upheaval, your requirements for magnesium escalate.[1, 2] Dr. Mildred Seelig felt that athletic adolescent boys and girls may need 7–10 mg/kg/day and pregnancy requirements should be a minimum of 450 mg a day or up to 15 mg/kg/day.[3] An average good diet may supply about 120 mg of magnesium per 1,000 calories, for an estimated daily intake of about 250 mg.[4, 5]

Since at best the body is actually absorbing only half of what is taken in, researchers feel that most people would benefit from magnesium supplementation. Otherwise, body tissue must be broken down to supply vital areas of the body with essential magnesium.[6, 7]

MAGNESIUM TESTING

You've heard the saying "To err is human, to forgive is divine"? In the medical world, to err is human, to test is divine.

Laboratory tests should be used to confirm what our senses and intuition tells us, but all too often doctors place all their faith in tests. Yet finding the definitive test for a condition, which can clinch a diagnosis, makes both doctor and patient feel safe. Over the years lab testing for minerals evolved from measurements done on whole blood to isolating minerals inside cells. The present state of the art, however, lies in testing mineral ions, which are the active component of minerals working at the tissue level. As mentioned throughout *The Magnesium Miracle*, much of the current research on magnesium has made use of ionic magnesium testing to measure magnesium at work in the cells; however, that testing is still not readily available to the public. A mineral measurement called EXATest and the red blood cell magnesium test, discussed below, provides readily available magnesium tests—although not as accurate as ionic magnesium testing, they are more accurate than serum magnesium tests.

There are two clinical tests that can be done in a doctor's office, the results of which can indicate both calcium deficiency and magnesium deficiency: Chvostek's sign (a contraction of the facial muscles caused by tapping lightly on the facial nerve located in front of the ear) and Trousseau's sign (a spasm of the hand muscles caused by applying a tourniquet or blood pressure cuff to the forearm below the elbow for three

minutes). But since neither test distinguishes calcium deficiency from magnesium deficiency, doctors use the tests to
only diagnose and treat calcium deficiency. As a result, if calcium supplements are recommended based on either of these
tests, magnesium levels are driven even lower, causing more
magnesium-deficiency symptoms.

SERUM (BLOOD) MAGNESIUM TEST

In spite of, or perhaps because of, all the metabolic processes
that rely on magnesium, less than 1 percent of our body's total
magnesium can be measured in our blood; the rest is busily oc-
cupied in the cells and tissues or holding our bones together.
Therefore, it is virtually impossible to make an accurate assessment of the level of magnesium in various body tissue cells
using a routine serum magnesium test. This test is often called
a total serum magnesium test, which you might imagine relates to all the magnesium in your body—but it does not.
Magnesium in the blood does not correlate with the amount of
magnesium in other parts of your body. In fact, if you are
under the stress of various ailments, your body pumps magnesium out of the cells and into the blood, giving the mistaken
appearance of normality on testing in spite of bodywide depletion. Unfortunately, most magnesium evaluations done in
hospitals and in laboratories use the antiquated serum magnesium test.

RED AND WHITE BLOOD CELL MAGNESIUM TESTS

All body cells, including red and white blood cells, contain
magnesium—up to 40 percent of the body's total. Because
red blood cells are 500 times more abundant in blood than
white blood cells, they are the preferred test material. Studies
show that blood cell magnesium is a much more accurate

measure of total body magnesium than the serum magnesium test. One study in childhood asthmatics compared serum magnesium levels to total white blood cell magnesium levels. While serum magnesium became elevated on the first day of an asthma attack, the white blood cell magnesium levels dropped dramatically, indicating the real state of affairs. As mentioned above, under stress magnesium is released from the cells, depleting them as it floods into the bloodstream.[8]

THE BUCCAL CELL SMEAR TEST (EXATest)

Using cells gently scraped from an area in the mouth between the bottom teeth and the back of the tongue provides an accurate means of measuring the amount of magnesium in the cells of the body. Measuring cellular magnesium in this way indicates the amount of magnesium in heart and muscle cells, the two major body tissues affected by magnesium deficiency.

The buccal cell smear test can be used to sample many things in cells; however, IntraCellular Diagnostics has developed a testing procedure called EXATest specifically to identify the amounts of certain minerals in the cell. The company sends sampling kits to your doctor's office, where a simple procedure, which takes about 60 seconds, is performed. Your doctor uses a wooden spatula to scrape off superficial layers of cells under your tongue. The scrapings are carefully placed on a microscope slide and sent back to the lab. A special electron microscope then measures the amount of magnesium and other minerals in the sample on the slide. The results are sent back to your doctor. Fortunately, the test is covered by Medicare and insurance companies.

For those who are curious about the details of the testing, an analytical scanning electron microscope with high-tech, computerized elemental X-ray analysis (EXA) bombards the specimen with high-energy electrons, whereupon energy is re-

orm of wavelengths that are distinct and unique
eral element. A computer measures the wave-
lengths and calculates what is called a "spectral fingerprint"
for each patient that identifies the mineral levels and ratios
within the cell. See the Resources section for IntraCellular Diagnostics contact information.

THE MAGNESIUM CHALLENGE TEST

Time-consuming and cumbersome but necessary for people
who may be magnesium wasters, the magnesium challenge
test requires twenty-four-hour urine collections on two separate occasions. The first urine collection is done when you are
taking your normal supplements. Then, in the doctor's office, a
dose of 2 meq/kg of magnesium chloride or magnesium sulfate is given intravenously, infused over a four-hour period. A
second urine collection begins after the IV, and every urine
sample is collected for twenty-four hours. Deficiency is diagnosed when the body exhibits a need for magnesium by holding
on to more than 25 percent of the magnesium given. A decade
ago, the magnesium challenge test was the best method of determining body stores.[9] While today comparison studies using
magnesium challenge and ionized magnesium indicate that
ionized magnesium testing appears to be a better indicator and
is more easily done (see next section),[10] the ionized magnesium
test is currently not available except for research purposes, so
the magnesium challenge test should be used.

The magnesium challenge test can diagnose magnesium
wasting. If more than 75 percent of the magnesium given in
the IV test is excreted, the assumption is that you have enough
magnesium and are not deficient. However, if a clinical assessment is made that you have magnesium deficiency symptoms
and you lose most of the magnesium given by IV, then magnesium wasting is the probable diagnosis. The treatment for

magnesium wasting is to take IV magnesium or use magnesium oil transdermal applications as described in Chapter 18.

BLOOD IONIZED MAGNESIUM TEST

The blood ionized magnesium test, pioneered and tested extensively at the State University of New York Downstate Medical Center in Brooklyn by magnesium researchers Bella and Burton Altura, is the most accurate and reliable magnesium blood test available but presently limited to research use. The Alturas have researched the health effects of magnesium since the 1960s and did the original research for the test in 1987.[11, 12, 13, 14, 15, 16]

The ionic magnesium test is a very refined procedure, backed up by results on many thousands of patients with over twenty-two different disease states and published in dozens of journals, including five papers in *Science* and papers in the prestigious *Scandinavian Journal of Clinical Laboratory Investigation* and *Scientific American*.[17] To determine the efficacy and efficiency of the new test, research included a comparison of magnesium levels found with the Alturas' ionized magnesium test to levels found in various body tissues using expensive and sensitive digital imaging microscopy, atomic absorption spectroscopy, and the magnesium fluorescent probe. The blood ionized magnesium test came through as a highly sensitive, convenient, and relatively inexpensive means of determining magnesium status in healthy or ill subjects.

Here's how it works. Magnesium exists in the body either as active magnesium ions bound to nothing or as inactive magnesium complexes (such as magnesium citrate) bound to proteins or other substances. A magnesium ion is an atom that is missing two electrons, which makes it search to attach to something that will replace its missing electrons. Magnesium ions constitute the physiologically active fraction of magnesium in the body; they are not attached to other substances and are free to join in biochemical body processes.[18]

Most clinical laboratories assess only *total* serum magnesium, which includes both active and inactive types. Since there is only 1 percent of the body's magnesium in the blood, however, the test samples only that 1 percent. With the blood ionized magnesium test it is now possible to directly measure the levels of magnesium ions in whole blood, plasma, and serum using ion-selective electrodes that gives an accurate accounting of the actual magnesium at work in the body.[19]

For example, ionized magnesium testing on 3,000 migraine patients shows that 90 percent of those with low magnesium ion levels improve with magnesium therapy. In 85 to 90 percent of all patients tested, low magnesium ion levels match tissue levels of free magnesium and accurately diagnose magnesium deficiency found in asthma, brain trauma, coronary artery disease, types I and II diabetes, gestational diabetes, eclampsia and preeclampsia, heart disease, homocysteinuria, hypertension, tension headaches, posttraumatic headaches, ischemic heart disease, liver transplant patients, renal transplant patients, polycystic ovarian disease, stroke, and syndrome X. In many of these conditions, low magnesium ion levels exist in spite of normal serum magnesium levels, making the ionized magnesium test more reliable for magnesium deficiency.[20, 21, 22, 23, 24, 25, 26, 27, 28, 29]

Because laboratories are slow to acquire new equipment, at present the FDA-approved ionized magnesium test is unfortunately mainly limited to the Alturas' laboratory and used mostly for research purposes. In the past, the Alturas have provided this test to doctors who sent in their patients' blood, but that avenue is less available now and few other labs are using the test. (See the Resources section for further information on the ionized magnesium test.)

THE ORAL CLINICAL TRIAL

For the average individual, one way to diagnose magnesium deficiency is simply to try supplementing. For one to three months take magnesium while recording all changes in your physical and mental health. It may be best to do this under a health professional's guidance, especially if you are on medications or have an existing medical condition. But we have long been our own caretakers and that freedom should not be taken from us. The alleviation of symptoms after thirty to ninety days constitutes the best proof that you had a magnesium deficiency. Adding magnesium oil or gel to your regimen can enhance the effects of oral supplementation. See pages 240–50 for types of magnesium and dosage.

FALSE-POSITIVE MAGNESIUM TESTS

The lack of adequate tools to measure magnesium in most hospitals and clinics is one of the main reasons medical doctors do not prescribe it. A serum magnesium test is actually worse than ineffective, because a test result that is within normal limits lends a false sense of security about the status of the mineral in the body. It also explains why doctors don't recognize magnesium deficiency; they assume serum magnesium levels are an accurate measure of all the magnesium in the body. Magnesium researchers also mostly use serum magnesium tests to determine magnesium status in their test subjects. As they begin to use the more accurate ionized magnesium test, however, the results will indicate even more widespread deficiency in the population.

===

CHAPTER SEVENTEEN

A MAGNESIUM EATING PLAN

Good nutrition creates a solid structural foundation of tissue and bone as well as nutrients for making hormones and neurotransmitters. The basis of good nutrition is the consumption of protein, minerals, trace minerals, vitamins, amino acids, and essential fatty acids. Clearly there is more to life than magnesium, but life can't exist without it. Just as important as magnesium is calcium, and the magnesium eating plan will also focus on how much calcium you need in your diet and in your supplement bottle.

The present American diet is heavily biased toward processed flour, sugar, and unhealthy fats. Over one-quarter of our diet may consist of what are in essence nonfoods that don't contain even a smattering of healthy nutrients. Magnesium is banished during food processing and never replaced, as some nutrients are, in fortified foods.

George Eby, whose foundation provided funds to educate members of Congress about magnesium and present them with copies of *The Magnesium Miracle*, has a personal interest in magnesium, having suffered from magnesium deficiency for many years. He is convinced that magnesium deficiency causes

50 to 70 percent of all our chronic illnesses and accounts for a huge share of medical and hospital expenses. He's also concerned that because most of us have grown up in a society with widespread magnesium deficiency, which began about 100 years ago with the large-scale refining of grain, we are unable to recognize that we are deficient. Eby says that white flour should be called not "refined" wheat but "depleted" wheat, and points to the November 2002 issue of the *Harvard Heart Letter*, which shows that only 16 percent of the magnesium remains after wheat is refined.

Eby reminds us that other critical nutrients, such as vitamins E and B_6, vital for proper absorption of magnesium, are also depleted by refining. However, magnesium is the main nutrient that is not adequately obtained by eating other foods. He says we are too fond of foods made with depleted wheat, such as pancakes, waffles, biscuits, tortillas, bread, cake, cookies, and doughnuts. These products take up a large amount of shelf space in grocery and convenience stores, mirroring our insatiable appetite for them. Clearly, he says, people love these foods—although a better verb would be *crave*, because people feel empty after eating depleted wheat, and keep eating more, perhaps searching for magnesium and other nutrients necessary for the body to function properly.

To obtain enough magnesium from the diet takes special care and knowledge of magnesium-rich foods, but we still need to supplement with magnesium. In 2005, Eby produced a DVD showing a long list of foods with the amounts necessary to deliver 400 mg of magnesium. Imagine 1.8 ounces of rice bran, which provides 400 mg of magnesium, beside 54.25 ounces of doughnuts, which is the quantity you have to eat to obtain the same amount of magnesium. Or visualize a few ounces of nuts compared to 25 ounces of white bread. Such a picture, showing the nutrient deficiency of refined foods, is worth a thousand words.

FOODS CONTAINING 400 MG OF MAGNESIUM
PER SERVING IN OUNCES

Food	Portion containing 400 mg
Rice bran, crude	1.8
Wheat bran, crude	2.3
Cocoa, dry powder	2.65
Pumpkin seeds	2.65
Brazil nuts	3.9
Peanut butter	3.9
Kellogg's All-Bran	3.9
Cashew nuts	4.80
Almonds	5.1
Quaker Oats	5.1
Baking chocolate	5.2
Molasses	5.3
Buckwheat flour	5.65
Oat bran	5.9
Wheat germ	5.9
Peanuts	8.0
Tortilla chips	14.5
Dinner rolls	16.6
Whole-wheat bread	17.3
English muffins	20
Potatoes	21.7
Spaghetti	22.0
Macaroni	22.0
Tortillas	22.0
Potato flour	22
Crackers	22.75
Melba toast	25
Bread, white	25
Potato chips	26
Brown sugar	48
Doughnuts	54.25

Statistics from USDA data

DIET SOLUTIONS TO MAGNESIUM DEFICIENCY

To enrich your diet with magnesium, increase your consumption of green vegetables, nuts, seeds, legumes, and unprocessed grains. Removing the germ and bran of cereals and further processing eliminates most of the magnesium present in the whole grain. It is a good idea to supplement a diet of vegetables, fruits, and protein-rich foods such as fish, meat, and milk by eating wheat germ, kelp, brewer's yeast, sunflower seeds, pumpkin seeds, and sea salt, which are all extremely rich in magnesium. Since one of the reasons you may be magnesium-deficient is from eating too much cooked and processed food, try to eat more raw foods. Fortunately, nuts, seeds, and many vegetables can be eaten raw, and raw wheat germ can be used on cereal and in protein drinks.

According to top French magnesium experts, highly effective heart- and blood-vessel-protective diets that reduce saturated fats, increase monounsaturated fat and omega-3 fatty acids (from fish and flaxseed), limit the consumption of alcohol, and increase the intake of cereals, fruits, vegetables, fish, and low-fat dairy products are rich in magnesium. They stress that among several protective nutrients, magnesium should be given particular consideration because of the very frequent occurrence of chronic primary magnesium deficiency, which acts as a cardiovascular risk factor.[1]

WHAT ABOUT CALCIUM?

As you can see from the list of calcium in common foods on pages 257–58, calcium is plentiful in nuts, seed, whole grains, and leafy green vegetables, just like magnesium, but only if the minerals are already in the soil. In theory, when you eat these foods you are getting a balanced amount of calcium and magnesium. Calcium is also found in seafood and dairy. So if you also eat these foods you shift the balance of calcium and magnesium in favor of calcium. Another important aspect of dietary calcium and magnesium is the effect of processing and cooking on these minerals. More magnesium is lost in food processing and cooking than calcium, so once again, more calcium is found in the diet than magnesium, which strengthens the case for taking magnesium in supplement form in equal amounts with calcium.

ORGANIC FOOD

Factory-farmed food is deficient in magnesium; therefore, organic food is a wiser choice. As more people go this route, whether to avoid herbicide and pesticide residues or to ensure nutrient-dense produce, the cost of organic food is dropping dramatically. However, organic food is not a guarantee of higher magnesium levels. Seek out organic farmers who are educated about crop rotation, test regularly for mineral deficiencies in the soil, and use mineral-rich fertilizers. The smart way to be assured of quality organic food is to join a community-sponsored agriculture (CSA) cooperative and buy a share in a local organic farm every year. Every week for an average of twenty-four weeks in the North, and all year round in the South, you share the harvest, which can include fresh vegetables, fruit, and free-range eggs, chicken, and lamb. (See the Resources section for information on CSAs.)

USDA FINDINGS

United States Department of Agriculture (USDA) surveys of women's diet find that approximately 25 percent of their magnesium is supplied by grain products. This means you should try to include a variety of whole grains and avoid white bread and pasta. If you crave sugar and bread, you may be feeding yeast in your intestines and should try to limit your intake to achieve weight loss and blood sugar balance. Or you may be craving nutrients that your body knows are absent from re-fined grains—you eat more carbs but the empty calories don't seem to satisfy a deeper need. Remember that you have to eat 25 ounces of white bread to get the RDA of magnesium.

Another 25 percent of women's magnesium intake comes from fruits and vegetables. The high-protein foods—meat, poul-try, and fish—provide only about 18 percent of total magne-sium intake. Since high-protein diets are now becoming more popular, you must make sure to increase your intake of mag-nesium when on such a diet. Fats, sweets, and beverages sup-ply 14 percent of the total magnesium intake; however, these foods, especially refined fats and sweets, should be limited be-cause they contain empty calories devoid of nutrients. Nuts and seeds and their butters are the richest sources of magne-sium, but they are not even mentioned in most food surveys.

FOODS RICH IN MAGNESIUM

In the Appendix you will find a complete list of foods with their magnesium content. Below is a short list of the richest sources of magnesium.[2] The quality of the soil from which these sources were assayed is unknown. Therefore, use these figures as a rough guide to making wise food choices.

MAGNESIUM CONTENT OF SELECTED FOODS

Food	Magnesium (mg) per 3½ oz (100 g/10 tbsp)
Kelp	760
Wheat Bran	490
Wheat germ	336
Almonds	270
Cashews	267
Molasses	258
Yeast, brewer's	231
Buckwheat	229
Brazil nuts	225
Dulse	220
Filberts	184
Peanuts	175
Wheat grain	160
Millet	162
Pecans	142
English walnuts	131
Rye	115
Tofu	111

HERB SOURCES OF MAGNESIUM

Green plants, including most herbs, such as purslane and cilantro, are loaded with magnesium.[3, 4, 5, 6] Here are some other commonly used magnesium-rich herbs that you can introduce into your diet. Herbs have the added advantage of often being organic or picked wild, so they usually don't contain pesticides and herbicides.

BURDOCK ROOT (ARCTIUM LAPPA), 537 MG MAGNESIUM PER 100 G

Master herbalist Matthew Wood describes burdock root as a natural diuretic specifically for flushing out very small kidney stones, an excellent blood cleanser, and a liver detoxifier. It can be grated into salads or cooked like potato and eaten several times per week.

CHICKWEED (*STELLARIA MEDIA*), 529 MG MAGNESIUM PER 100 G

Herbalist Susun Weed describes chickweed as a perfect food with "optimum nutrition." Chickweed encourages absorption of minerals and nutrients and is also naturally high in magnesium. Used several times a week in salads, it provides an excellent source of dietary magnesium.

DANDELION (*TARAXACUM OFFICINALE*), 157 MG MAGNESIUM PER 100 G

This amazing herb has been vilified as a nuisance weed, but its healing properties are legion. According to Andrew Chevallier, an experienced medical herbalist, it is used as a safe, natural diuretic to treat high blood pressure, and as a detoxifier to remove waste products from the gallbladder and the kidneys, thereby ameliorating many conditions such as gallstones, constipation, acne, eczema, arthritis, and gout. No doubt it owes some of its actions to the properties of magnesium. Dandelion leaves, used in salads, add a necessary bitter property that stimulates the bile. The root can be cooked or grated raw into salads.

DULSE (*PALMARIA PALMATA*), 220 MG MAGNESIUM PER 100 G

Dulse is a type of seaweed, of which there are many kinds; all dietary seaweeds are very nutritious. They are very high in digestible protein, around 25 percent by weight. Iodine to support the thyroid gland is their most notable benefit. They are high in most minerals as well as vitamins. Dulse can be introduced several times a week in soups and stews, and don't forget vegetarian sushi rolls, which are wrapped in seaweed.

**NETTLES (*URTICA DIOICA*), 860 MG MAGNESIUM
PER 100 G**

Nettles are used to soften gallstones or kidney stones in the body. Susun Weed has some excellent recipes for nettles in her book *Healing Wise*. When nettles are lightly steamed they lose their stinging properties and make an excellent vegetable addition to any meal.

MAGNESIUM SALT SUBSTITUTES

Most doctors tell patients with high blood pressure to avoid salt, but they mean sodium chloride. Salt from the sea and salt high in magnesium are not only safe but can be therapeutic for someone with heart disease. They do contain sodium, however, so be sure to read labels.

Celtic Sea Salt is all the rage in gourmet food shops and it should be in your kitchen and dining room as well. Salt from evaporated seawater is relatively high in magnesium and is a wonderful way to get extra magnesium—about 20 mg in a teaspoon. However, the sodium content is still excessively high.

Smart Salt is just that—a smart way to stock up on magnesium. Smart Salt is a product of the United States, produced by evaporation from Utah's Great Salt Lake. It has the following levels of minerals in 3 tsp: 626 mg of magnesium, 865 mg of potassium, and only 1,596 mg of sodium. (A similar amount of table salt contains about 5,000 mg of sodium.)

Cardia Salt offers a healthy combination of salt, potassium, and magnesium that tastes just like regular salt. It produced a reduction in blood pressure in a double-blind placebo-controlled study carried out in 1997 on 233 hypertensive patients on medication. Another half dozen studies have confirmed its safety and effectiveness. Researchers comment that the product works because it reduces the amount of sodium by 50 percent and raises potassium and magnesium levels. For every teaspoon of salt you net about 40 mg of magnesium. The average amount of salt used per day is about 3 tsp, which means a significant 120 mg of magnesium per day, but, again, the sodium levels are still very high compared to magnesium. See the Resources section for magnesium salt substitutes.

MINERAL WATER AND MAGNESIUM

An important source of magnesium, popular in Europe, is magnesium-rich mineral water. We have only a few local waters in the United States that have high magnesium levels that could help to reduce magnesium deficiency. We must also be careful to consider the calcium content of bottled water in relation to magnesium. A close reading of mineral water labels tells us that the calcium and sodium content is usually much higher than magnesium. Therefore, choose water with calcium no more than twice the level of magnesium. This will ensure that you are getting enough of both minerals. If, however, you know you have a magnesium deficiency, by symptoms or by medical or naturopathic diagnosis, choose water with high magnesium and low calcium content for replacement. And if you suffer from heart disease, choose mineral water that also has a low sodium content. Be aware that even though a label says "mineral water," the mineral content may be minuscule and not worth the price you pay.[7]

Another important aspect of drinking water that I discuss with clients in my telephone consulting practice is whether it is acid or alkaline. Our bodies are 70–90 percent water, so finding ways to increase the alkalinity of the body is vital to health.

MAGNESIUM IN WATER[8]

Water Name	Country	Magnesium (mg/L)	Calcium (mg/L)	Sodium (mg/L)
Adobe Springs	USA	96	3.3	5
Santa Ynez	USA	87	19	—
San Pellegrino	Italy	57	203	46
Penafiel	Mexico	41	131	159
Vittel	France	38	181	3.7
Evian	France	24	78	5
Naya	Canada	22	38	6
Volvic	France	7	10	10.7
Saratoga	USA	7	64	9
Perrier	France	5	143	15.2
Alhambra	USA	5	9.5	5.4
Arrowhead	USA	5	20	3
Sparkletts	USA	5	4.6	15.2
Calistoga	USA	2	8	163
Cobb Mountain	USA	2	5.6	4.6
Poland Spring	USA	2	13.2	8.9
Sante	USA	1	4.2	160
Black Mountain	USA	1	25	8.3
Crystal Geyser	USA	1	1.5	30

A MAGNESIUM EATING PLAN

Upon rising: Juice of ½–1 fresh lemon in warm water. Sweeten with stevia.

BREAKFAST

Crockpot cereal with flaxseed oil and fresh or frozen blueberries, strawberries, raspberries, banana, peach, or pear

Choose two grains, one nut, one seed from: buckwheat, millet, rye, oats, amaranth, quinoa, sunflower seeds, pumpkin seeds, almonds, cashews, filberts, walnuts, pecans

For one person, put 2 oz of dry mixture in 5 oz of water in a 1-quart crockpot. Cook overnight. In the morning place in a bowl, add 2–4 oz of fruit, mix, and add 2 tbsp flaxseed oil *or* 1 tbsp butter (organic), *or* 2 tbsp ground flaxseeds (ground fresh in a coffee grinder). You may add rice milk, almond milk, or small amounts of soy milk as needed. For extra magnesium, sprinkle on wheat germ (kept in the freezer).

Substitutions:

1. Instead of using a crockpot, you can soak 2 oz of grain mixture overnight in 5 oz of water, with or without 2 tbsp of plain yogurt. In the morning bring to a boil and let simmer on the lowest setting for 20 minutes. You may have to add more water to avoid dryness. Serve with 2 tbsp ground flaxseeds (ground fresh in a coffee grinder).

2. Instead of soaking overnight, cook 2 oz of grain mixture in 6 oz of water. Bring to a boil and let simmer for 30 minutes.

LUNCH (*Choose one*)

Brown rice and vegetables, cooked with 2 oz dulse or other sea vegetables

Leafy green salad, soup with added sea vegetables,
and Essene sprouted bread or Ezekiel bread

Fish, greens (collards, spinach, swiss chard), and
salad

Egg omelet with sautéed vegetables

Chicken with vegetables

DINNER (*Choose one*)

Soup (with sea vegetables) and salad

Stir-fried grains (leftover grains from breakfast) and
vegetables

Roasted vegetables with wild rice

Salad with cooked organic legumes (kidney beans,
lentils, black beans, pinto beans, chickpeas)

Wheat-free pasta (rice, spelt, kamut) with pesto,
tomato sauce, and green vegetables

Mixed salad with avocado

SNACKS

Raw vegetables

Dried fruit (prunes and figs)

Shelled nuts and seeds (raw, not processed or salted)

Baked blue corn chips

Popcorn

DRINKS

Pure, clean water

Green tea

Freshly squeezed lemon juice and water

Cranberry juice sweetened with stevia

Herbal teas

Kukicha (roasted twig tea)

THE MAGNESIUM DIET

- Eat a wide variety of vegetables daily. Always include greens such as kale, collards, spinach, and curly-leaf lettuce, and magnesium-rich herbs such as dandelion, chickweed, and nettles.
- Enjoy starchy vegetables three or four times a week, such as red-skinned potatoes, winter squash, corn on the cob, lima beans, and burdock root.
- Eat fruits moderately.
- Include a variety of whole grains: buckwheat, millet, rye, oats, amaranth, and quinoa.
- Fish, shellfish, organic chicken, meat, turkey, or free-range eggs can be eaten once a day as rich animal protein sources.
- Have beans, tempeh, nuts, seeds, and legumes as a vegetarian source of protein daily.
- Use fresh and dry herbs in your cooking and include lots of garlic.
- Use organic cold-pressed oils for your cooking: extra-virgin olive oil, coconut oil, and sesame oil.
- Use organic butter in moderation.
- Take 1–2 tbsp of flaxseed oil daily.
- Use whole-grain breads and pasta.
- For sweetener use stevia.
- Drink natural spring, distilled, or filtered water only.
- Enjoy organic herbal teas.
- Eat sea vegetables: dulse, nori, arame, wakame, kombu, and hijiki. All are exceedingly high in magnesium.
- Use natural raw, unheated nuts, seeds, and nut and seed butters, rich magnesium sources.
- Use a high-quality mineral-rich sea salt.

FOODS TO AVOID (READ LABELS THOROUGHLY)

- All refined and processed foods of any kind, such as cookies, cakes, doughnuts, bagels, white bread, luncheon meats, and soy protein powder.
- All refined and processed sugars, including fructose or corn syrup and diet products with artificial sweeteners such as aspartame (NutraSweet and Splenda).
- All dairy products except organic butter and free-range eggs.
- Regular and decaffeinated coffee or black tea.
- Any foods containing hydrogenated or partially hydrogenated oils or trans fatty acids.
- All alcoholic beverages.
- Pasteurized fruit juices and sodas.
- Foods containing MSG, hydrolyzed vegetable protein, and chemical preservatives.
- Commercial iodized salt.

CHAPTER EIGHTEEN

MAGNESIUM SUPPLEMENTATION AND HOMEOPATHIC MAGNESIUM

When you take supplements it can be a real challenge to find out how much actual or elemental magnesium is available in each pill or capsule and even harder to find out how much you need. Magnesium does not exist alone in nature but comes combined with other substances. That other substance, tagging along with magnesium, has a specific weight. For example, 1,000 mg of magnesium citrate, the mostly commonly used form of magnesium, offers 125 mg of elemental magnesium. When reading the label, the amount of elemental magnesium is what you want. The best forms of magnesium are magnesium taurate, magnesium glycinate, magnesium citrate, magnesium malate, magnesium orotate, and magnesium oil.

There is one more thing to be aware of on product labels, which is the specification of dosage. All too often people will find that they have to take not one but three or six tablets to make up the dosage on the label. It may be in small print, but read it carefully to understand exactly what each tablet contains.

MAGNESIUM DOSAGE

To individualize your magnesium dosage, the rule of thumb for men is 6–8 mg/kg (3.0 to 4.5 mg/lb) of body weight per day. That translates into a total dietary and supplemental magnesium of 600 to 900 mg per day for a 200-lb man. Some researchers recommend 10 mg/kg/day for children because of their low body weight and increased requirements for growth and 6–10 mg/kg/day for athletes, depending on stress and training levels.[1, 2, 3, 4]

CONTRAINDICATIONS TO MAGNESIUM THERAPY

1. *Kidney failure.* With kidney failure there is an inability to clear magnesium from the kidneys.
2. *Myasthenia gravis.* Intravenous administration could accentuate muscle relaxation and collapse the respiratory muscles.
3. *Excessively slow heart rate.* Slow heart rates can be made even slower, as magnesium relaxes the heart. Slow heart rates often require an artificial pacemaker.
4. *Bowel obstruction.* The main route of elimination of oral magnesium is through the bowel.

THE SAFETY OF MAGNESIUM SUPPLEMENTS

For the average person, oral magnesium, even in high dosages, has no side effects except loose stools, which is a mechanism to release excess magnesium and an indication to cut back. Excess magnesium is also lost through the urine.

TYPES OF MAGNESIUM

ORAL SUPPLEMENTS

Bone meal is a rich source of magnesium. More than 60 percent of the magnesium in the bodies of humans and animals is in the bones and teeth. However, since 1945, radioactive strontium 90, along with lead and a variety of other toxic elements, began to show up in our bones and in the bones of cattle, from which bone meal is produced. It is important, therefore, to find an organic source of bone meal, strictly assayed for contaminants, if you wish to consume this product. Another reason it makes good sense to use only organic animal products is the threat of mad cow disease.

When you look at the amount of elemental magnesium in various supplements, you see that magnesium oxide seems to have a higher amount of available magnesium; however, recent studies have shown that only about 4 percent of that amount is absorbed. We are told that about 50 percent of magnesium in foods and water is absorbed. All other supplements range somewhere in between.

Chelated magnesium, bound to organic amino acids, is far better absorbed than magnesium oxide but is more expensive. Complementary medicine practitioners rely on chelated magnesium, such as magnesium glycinate, taurate, and orotate, to treat serious cases of magnesium deficiency. Dr. Russell Blaylock warns that magnesium aspartate may offer the body too much aspartic acid, an amino acid that causes brain stimulation; he recommends avoidance.

Weight for weight and dollar for dollar, *magnesium citrate* may be the best buy for general use. It is probably the mostly widely used magnesium supplement because it's inexpensive, easily absorbed, and only has a mild laxative effect. The best form is a magnesium citrate powder mixed in water that can be taken every day. However, if you walk into your average pharmacy and ask for magnesium citrate, you will be directed, usually in a loud voice, to bowel-purging laxatives. I learned about citrate salts in medical school; in large amounts they are used to completely purge the bowel before bowel X-rays, barium enemas, sigmoidoscopies, or colonoscopies. For example, the total amount taken daily as a magnesium citrate supplement is about 900 mg. However, 12,000 mg is the amount given for a bowel purge! If your pharmacist doesn't know the difference between a magnesium citrate supplement and a bowel-purging laxative, just go down the street and find a health food store, which is sure to have magnesium citrate in powder as well as capsules.

FORMS OF MAGNESIUM

Inorganic salts	Organic salt chelates
Magnesium bicarbonate	Dimagnesium malate
Magnesium carbonate	Magnesium adipate
Magnesium chloride	Magnesium aspartate
Magnesium oxide	Magnesium citrate
Magnesium phosphate	Magnesium glutamate
Magnesium sulfate	Magnesium glycinate
	Magnesium lysinate
	Magnesium malate
	Magnesium orotate
	Magnesium taurate

MAGNESIUM CONTENT OF VARIOUS SUPPLEMENTS

Magnesium Salt	Amount of Elemental Magnesium per 500 mg Salt
Magnesium oxide	300 mg
Magnesium carbonate	150 mg
Dimagnesium malate	95 mg
Dolomite	75 mg
Magnesium citrate	75 mg
Magnesium malate	75 mg
Magnesium chloride	60 mg
Magnesium lactate	60 mg
Magnesium glycinate	50 mg
Magnesium sulfate	50 mg
Magnesium taurate	50 mg
Magnesium orotate	30 mg
Magnesium gluconate	25 mg

MAGNESIUM SUPPLEMENT ABSORPTION

The amount of magnesium your tissues can readily use is based on how soluble the magnesium product is and the amount of elemental or ionic magnesium that is released. A value, called a stability constant, is placed on all metal-ligand complexes. Magnesium citrate is a metal-ligand complex; the metal is magnesium and the ligand is citric acid. Magnesium taurate is a metal-ligand complex composed of the metal magnesium and the ligand taurine. Stability constants range from less than one into the teens. If a metal-ligand has a very low stability constant (less than 1), the metal-ligand is readily soluble in water and also easily dissociates into the metal ionic form shown and the ligand. This means your body is able to absorb the metal ingested in ionic form at a pH as low as stomach acid (about pH 2 to 3) to as high as pH 7.4, which is the pH of the main extracellular body fluids such as serum and lymph.

There are three ranges of stability constants and absorption.

- Metal-ligand complexes with stability constants of 3 and lower are soluble and substantially ionized at physiologic pH 7.4.
- Metal-ligand complexes with stability constants over 3 and perhaps as high as 6 are likely to disassociate in stomach acid, but not greatly at physiologic pH 7.4.
- Metal-ligand complexes with stability constants above 6 release less metal regardless of how low the pH may be, and such compounds are essentially useless in biological systems.

To simplify this complex system, in order for minerals to be biologically available for human and animal use, they should not be associated with ligands where the stability constant is greater than 4.0.

The stability constants of amino acid complexes of many biologically important metals are in the 3 to 4 range and are highly absorbed even though they are not necessarily broken down by acids.

Magnesium Complex	Stability Constant	Ionization
Magnesium chloride	0	(totally ionized)
Magnesium acetate	0.51	(essentially ionized)
Magnesium gluconate	0.70	(essentially ionized)
Magnesium lactate	0.93	(essentially ionized)
Magnesium malate	1.55	(essentially ionized)
Magnesium glutamate*	1.90	(essentially ionized but neurotoxic)

*Avoid magnesium glutamate; it breaks down into the neurotransmitter glutamic acid, which without being bound to other amino acids is neurotoxic. Glutamic acid is a component of aspartame, which should also be avoided.

Magnesium aspartate*	2.43	(essentially ionized but neurotoxic)
Magnesium citrate	2.8	essentially ionized
Magnesium glycinate	3.45	

*Avoid this form; it breaks down into the neurotransmitter aspartic acid, which without being bound to other amino acids is neurotoxic. Aspartic acid is a component of aspartame, which also should be avoided.

Reference: george-eby-research.com/html/stability_constants.html. Note: On this site taurine is not listed, and orotic acid does not have a stability constant associated with magnesium, so they were not included.

Magnesium taurate, glycinate, and orotate are amino acid chelates of magnesium that have less laxative effect on the intestines than magnesium citrate, so they are recommended if you tend to have loose stools. Magnesium taurate is a combination of the amino acid taurine and magnesium that has special properties for the heart. Taken together in this combination, magnesium and taurine have a synergistic effect, stabilizing cell membranes, calming the nervous system, and inhibiting nerve excitation. Taurine also transports magnesium across cell membranes, making this form of magnesium highly absorbed. Magnesium taurate does not have a great laxative effect and is the recommended form of magnesium for people with heart problems. In a series of studies published since the early 1970s it appears that the amino acid taurine is important for heart health and may prevent arrythmias and protect the heart against the damage caused by heart attacks.[5, 6]

Magnesium chloride is a form of magnesium that comes in

capsules, powder, and IV solution. Some researchers say it may be the best form of magnesium for ingestion, because minerals need to be dissolved in acid before they can go into solution. Magnesium chloride has enough extra chloride to produce hydrochloric acid in the stomach to enhance its absorption. In the stomach, there is normally sufficient hydrochloric acid present, but if you take a lot of antacid products, the chemical conversion can be compromised.

Dr. José Luis Pérez Albela, director of the Instituto Bien de Salud in Lima, Peru, is an ardent proponent of magnesium and uses magnesium chloride exclusively. He spreads the word on his radio show, in public lectures, to his colleagues, and to his patients. He manufactures and distributes small one-dose packets of magnesium chloride, often giving them away to needy people. To overcome the bitter taste, he tells people to stir the powder in citrus juice. Or you can put a drop of lemon or orange essential oil in a glass of water and stir in the powder. Success stories with magnesium from Dr. Albela's patients and friends could fill a book. Magnesium chloride is the form of magnesium used to make magnesium oil.

Magnesium malate combines magnesium with malic acid, a weak organic acid found in vegetables and fruit, especially apples. The weak bond with magnesium makes it readily soluble in the body. Malic acid is a key component of several energy-making chemical reactions in the body. Researchers have used magnesium malate successfully to treat the chronic fatigue, pain, and insomnia of fibromyalgia. Dimagnesium malate increases the amount of magnesium available to the body; it has the same properties as magnesium malate.

Magnesium oxide appears to have a high amount of elemental magnesium. One 500-mg capsule of magnesium oxide contains 300 mg of elemental magnesium. But little of that amount is available to the body because it is not absorbed and therefore not biologically available. One recent study reported a 4 percent absorption rate of magnesium oxide. This means 12 mg of a 500 mg capsule are absorbed and 288 mg stay in the intestines, acting like a laxative. Most of the medical research done on magnesium employs magnesium oxide. Imagine how much more favorable the results would be if a more absorbable form of magnesium were used.

There are several ways to enhance absorption besides choosing an absorbable product. If you have digestive problems with symptoms of gas and bloating, which indicates a lack of hydrochloric acid, you may need to take a digestive aid such as betaine hydrochloride to help absorb your minerals. Magnesium can be taken with or without meals, but it's preferable to take it between meals for better absorption. Magnesium requires stomach acid to be absorbed. After a full meal, your stomach acid is busy digesting food and may not be available to help absorb the magnesium. Also, magnesium is an alkaline mineral and acts like an antacid; taken with meals, it may neutralize stomach acid and impair digestion.

If you develop loose stools while taking magnesium, it does not necessarily mean you are absorbing enough and losing the rest; it may mean you are taking too much at one time. Never take your daily magnesium all at once. Spread it out through the day; four times a day is best if you've been experiencing diarrhea. If that doesn't do the trick, you probably need to cut back the amount you're taking or switch to another type or brand of magnesium. Taking magnesium oil for at least half your daily supplement will often banish loose stools.

Remember that when you first begin taking magnesium, you may need a high amount to remedy an existing deficiency, but over time that deficiency will be eliminated and you might need less. Your stools will tell you. *Note:* If you are taking a multivitamin-mineral supplement, remember to check the amount of elemental magnesium on the label and count it in your daily total. And if you follow the magnesium eating plan

7, the extra magnesium in your diet means you
ss in supplement form.

MAGNESIUM OIL

A very exciting addition to the magnesium family is a product loosely referred to as magnesium oil. It's not actually an oil at all, but a supersaturated solution of magnesium chloride in water. Magnesium oil can be sprayed or rubbed on the body and is readily absorbed through the skin. It helps greatly to increase the amount of magnesium in body tissues and overcomes the problems that some people have with loose stools when they try to take enough magnesium to meet their needs. This can be especially important in cases of severe magnesium deficiency that were treatable only with IV magnesium before magnesium oil came along.

Norman Shealy, M.D., Ph.D., neurosurgeon and world-renowned pain management expert, confirms that sufficient magnesium is notoriously difficult to absorb orally when it acts like a laxative. He says that if magnesium goes through the intestines in less than twelve hours, absorption of the mineral is seriously impaired. It's excreted faster than it can be absorbed. Dr. Shealy is also convinced that even the best oral preparation, which he considers to be magnesium taurate, requires oral supplementation for six to twelve months to restore intracellular levels. But he finds that skin application of magnesium oil with a concentration of 25 percent magnesium chloride restores intracellular levels within four to six weeks. Dr. Shealy has produced a small study to support his findings.

According to Mark Sircus, O.M.D., who writes about magnesium oil in *Transdermal Magnesium Therapy* (Phaelos Books, 2006), the amount of magnesium in one spray of a 25 or 35 percent solution of magnesium chloride is between 13 and 18 mg. Therefore, if you pump about 6 sprays for each leg and arm, you are applying about 400 mg of magnesium—the

RDA. Another 6 sprays to your front and 6 to your back and you have a 600 mg dosage. If the magnesium oil tingles or burns slightly, you can dilute the oil by pouring out half the bottle into another container and filling the spray bottle with distilled water. This cuts the dosage in half, so you need to use twice as many sprays to get 600 mg. After about thirty minutes, most of the magnesium has already been absorbed, so if the oil feels a bit itchy when it dries, you can wash it off in a quick shower, or just simply wash the itchy areas with a washcloth.

MAGNESIUM SHOTS

In her book *Diagnosing and Treating Chronic Fatigue Syndrome,* English doctor Sarah Mayhill gives a good account of the administration of magnesium by intravenous (IV) and intramuscular (IM) shots. Dr. Mayhill uses 2 ml, which is about half a teaspoon, of 50 percent magnesium sulfate, equal to only 100 mg of elemental magnesium, by IM or IV injection every two weeks to keep the levels up in her chronic fatigue patients. Such a shot, into muscle, can be painful. It is given slowly over one to two minutes. It goes directly into the bloodstream through small capillaries and can make you feel hot, flushed, and anxious, as it causes a generalized dilation of all the blood vessels in the body, but this is in no way harmful.

Intravenous magnesium should be used immediately at the onset of a heart attack or stroke. These conditions are due to a blockage and spasm of arteries, and the vasodilation produced is extremely beneficial. The dosage is 2–5 ml of 50 percent magnesium sulfate injected directly into a vein. The amount of elemental magnesium in this dose is 100–250 mg. Most clinical trials using magnesium offer this dose.

Magnesium oxide, hydroxide, and carbonate are not soluble and not bioavailable and only very slightly bioavailable. They act mainly as laxatives, leaving almost no magnesium to be absorbed. If you take a magnesium tablet or capsule and get loose stools, then you know it's not being absorbed but sweeping through your intestines, pushing everything along with it.

IV magnesium is the most absorbable form of magnesium, and magnesium oil is the second best. Third best are the oral forms magnesium glycinate, magnesium taurate, and magnesium orotate. Fourth comes magnesium citrate, but since it's usually cheaper than other oral forms, it's become the most popular. Magnesium oxide is a distinct fifth and very poorly absorbed, but it makes a great laxative.

WHEN TO TAKE MAGNESIUM

Take your first dose of magnesium when you wake up in the morning and the last dose at bedtime. If you take a third dose, make it late in the afternoon. Magnesium is most deficient in the early morning and late afternoon. A very few people feel that magnesium is sufficiently energizing that it keeps them awake at night, but most people find it as good as a sleeping pill to help them get a good night's rest. Others, who suffer from leg cramps, restless legs, fibromyalgia, or general muscle tension, take magnesium at night and find that it diminishes pain and tension and helps them sleep. There are so many ways that magnesium can work on the body that it is important for you to decide what timing is best for you.

MAGNESIUM AS A LAXATIVE

Oral doses of magnesium sulfate (Epsom salts), magnesium hydroxide (milk of magnesia), magnesium oxide, and magnesium citrate contain high concentrations of magnesium to draw water into the colon and act as an effective laxative. But it's all a matter of dose. As a laxative, 1,000–2,000 mg of milk of magnesia provides an effective dose; however, as a magnesium supplement, doses of 200–600 mg are more common.

These salts are, in fact, gentler than cascara and senna, herbs that cause muscle contraction of the intestinal wall. In *IBS for Dummies* (Dean and Wheeler, 2005), we talk about magnesium as an excellent treatment for IBS constipation as a daily supplement to prevent the problem from occurring.

Laxatives, in general, are not recommended because you can become dependent on them and they can flush out beneficial intestinal bacteria and electrolytes. It is far better to supplement the diet with magnesium-rich foods and, if necessary, magnesium supplements to relax the bowel and allow normal action. Magnesium laxatives are contraindicated in patients with nausea, vomiting, appendicitis, intestinal obstruction, undiagnosed abdominal pain, or kidney disease.

Epsom salts in a bath are absorbed slightly and are known to be relaxing. I remember one patient, Arlene, as "the woman who soaked too long." She put several pounds of Epsom salts in a bath, soaked for two hours, and found out that magnesium sulfate is indeed absorbed through the skin: she developed diarrhea due to magnesium's laxative effect. Someone with a skin condition such as eczema might absorb magnesium even more readily. Limit your soak to thirty minutes and follow the directions on the label for how much Epsom salts to add to your bath (as a general rule, use no more than 2 cups at a time).

CALCIUM AND MAGNESIUM INTERACTION

Watch your calcium intake. We know that too much calcium will impede magnesium uptake and function. Push aside the media-generated hype on calcium and look at the facts. A thousand years ago our diet favored magnesium over calcium. Now, however, we tend to get far more calcium in our diets than magnesium. Current research seems to indicate that two parts calcium to one part magnesium is probably most beneficial, with average optimal amounts of calcium at 1,000 mg per day and magnesium at 600 mg, which includes diet and supplementation.[7]

If you have definite magnesium deficiency symptoms, however, you may want to take even more magnesium—at least equal amounts of calcium and magnesium or even twice the amount of magnesium to calcium until your symptoms abate. If you do take too much magnesium, the only sign will be increased bowel movements as it flushes out of the body. As mentioned above, if you can't seem to get enough magnesium without having loose stools, then add magnesium oil to your regimen.

MAGNESIUM'S INTERACTION WITH OTHER NUTRIENTS

Magnesium is extremely important for the metabolism of calcium, potassium, phosphorus, zinc, copper, iron, sodium, lead, cadmium, hydrochloric acid, acetylcholine, and nitric oxide, as well as for the activation of vitamin B_1 and therefore for a very wide spectrum of crucial body functions.[8] A shift in any one of these nutrients has an impact on magnesium levels and vice versa. It is the interwoven nature of the body's components that makes it so difficult to isolate one substance to scientifically "prove" what it can do. Magnesium cannot be taken out of context either in a research setting or in your body. For example, you should increase magnesium intake when you consume more phosphorus and vitamin D. Magnesium is necessary to convert dietary vitamin D into one of the hormones that makes efficient use of calcium in bone formation.[9, 10] Vitamin B_6 increases the amount of magnesium that can enter cells; as a result, these two nutrients are often taken together. In one experiment, serum vitamin E levels improved after magnesium supplementation.[11] We also know that magnesium and the essential fatty acids (EFAs, found in fish, nuts and seeds, and flaxseed oil) are interdependent; each works much more efficiently when the other is present in sufficient amounts.

HOMEOPATHIC MAGNESIUM: ANOTHER FORM OF MAGNESIUM

Developed by Samuel Hahneman in the early nineteenth century, homeopathy is a natural medical science that uses mostly plants and mineral extracts diluted in alcohol or water to infinitesimal amounts in order to stimulate the individual's natural healing response. Research has shown that these substances, if given in a toxic amount, can cause symptoms similar to those that the patient is experiencing, but that the infinitesimal dose can cure those symptoms. After two hundred years of clinical use and observation, homeopathy is now more successful than the tools we have available to measure how it works. Although skeptics often attribute its success to the placebo effect, in which a patient's belief in an outcome produces that outcome, the millions who have benefited from homeopathy include infants and animals, two groups that are clearly not susceptible to the placebo effect.

Nonetheless, in America homeopathy continues to be marginalized in favor of other drugs, even in the face of such early evidence as the influenza epidemic of 1919, in which the homeopathic hospitals in England showed a greater cure rate than conventional hospitals. In Europe, both homeopathic medicine and herbal medicine enjoy a respected place in the health care system.

Homeopathic remedies typically come in dosages of 6, 12, or 30 X (10) or C (100) potency. The higher the number, the greater the dilution and the more potent the remedy. Usually, you take three pellets or four drops of a remedy several times a day. For a very acute, painful symptom, a dose can be taken every fifteen minutes. However, if after taking five or six doses of a remedy there is no change in symptoms, the remedy is probably ineffective and you should seek a new one. Be assured that treating with the wrong remedy a half dozen times does not cause any negative side effects.

In homeopathy, magnesium is used primarily for acute muscle spasms or chronic complaints.[12] Please consult a homeopath for a more detailed evaluation of your case.

Magnesia phosphorica (magnesium phosphate, or mag phos) is a great antispasmodic remedy and the most commonly used magnesium homeopathic remedy. It readily treats cramping of all muscles, including hiccups, leg cramps, writer's cramp, abdominal colic, heart pain, lung pain, menstrual pain accompanied by radiating pains, neuralgic pains, and all sorts of tics and tremors including twitching of the eyelids. It works especially well in debilitated subjects who are both mentally and physically tired.

Dr. Margery Mullins, an internist and acupuncturist, told me about the success she has had with the use of magnesium phosphate for muscle spasms with her patients. She said patients would get instant relief and then didn't seem to need the remedy after their magnesium deficiency was corrected with diet and supplements. One of her young patients, a nine-year-old girl, was having such severe muscle spasms that she was referred to a pediatric neurologist. In the interim, Dr. Mullins gave her Magnesia phosphorica 6X, and by the time of her appointment with the specialist the child no longer had the problem. Dr. Mullins noted that the girl's mother had had toxemia (eclampsia) during her pregnancy, requiring intravenous magnesium.

APPENDIX

MAGNESIUM CONTENT OF COMMON FOODS

Food	Magnesium (mg) per 3½ oz (100g) serving
Kelp	760
Wheat bran	490
Wheat germ	336
Almonds	270
Cashews	267
Molasses	258
Yeast, brewer's	231
Buckwheat	229
Brazil nuts	225
Dulse	220
Filberts	184
Peanuts	175
Millet	162
Wheat grain	160
Pecan	142
English walnuts	131
Rye	115

Food	Magnesium (mg) per 3 1/2 oz (100g) serving
Tofu	111
Coconut meat, dried	90
Brown rice	88
Soybeans, cooked	88
Figs, dried	71
Apricots	62
Dates	58
Collard greens	57
Shrimp	51
Corn, sweet	48
Avocado	45
Cheddar cheese	45
Parsley	41
Prunes, dried	40
Sunfower seeds	38
Barley	37
Beans, cooked	37
Dandelion greens	36
Garlic	36
Raisins	35
Green peas, fresh	35
Potato with skin	34
Crab	34
Banana	33
Sweet potato	31
Blackberry	30
Beets	25
Broccoli	24
Cauliflower	24
Carrot	23
Celery	22
Beef	21
Asparagus	20

Food	Magnesium (mg) per 3 1/2 oz (100g) serving
Chicken	19
Green pepper	18
Winter squash	17
Cantaloupe	16
Eggplant	16
Tomato	14
Milk	13

CALCIUM CONTENT OF COMMON FOODS

Food	Mg Calcium
Vegetables	
½ cup cooked spinach	88
1 cup cooked dried beans (white, kidney, soy, and so on)	95–110
½ cup cooked kale	103
½ cup cooked collards	110
1 cup cooked turnip greens	126
½ cup cooked dandelion greens	147
½ cup cooked beet greens	157
1 medium stalk broccoli	158
1 cup bok choy (Chinese cabbage)	252
Baked Goods and Ingredients	
1 slice whole-wheat bread	50
1 medium waffle	76
1 medium corn muffin	96
½ cup soy flour	132
1 tablespoon blackstrap molasses	140

Seafood

¾ 8-oz can clams	62
6 scallops	115
½ 7-oz can salmon with bones	284
20 medium oysters	300
7 sardines with bones	393

Nuts and Seeds

½ cup sesame seeds	76
½ cup Brazil nuts	128
½ cup almonds	175

Fruit

½ cup cooked rhubarb	200

Taken from *Natural Prescriptions for Common Ailments* (McGraw-Hill, 2001)

RESOURCES

MAGNESIUM PRODUCTS

Updated information on safe and effective magnesium products can be found by consulting Dr. Dean at www.carolyndean .com, as well as by private, customized consultations by phone and e-mail.

RELOX PROCEDURE

Dr. Bruce Rind and Dr. Sean Dalton
National Integrated Health Associates
5225 Wisconsin Avenue, Suite 401
Washington DC 20015
(202) 237-7000
Fax (202) 237-0017
www.drrind.com
Educational videos available online

T SUBSTITUTES

Nutrition 21
4 Manhattanville Road
Purchase, NY 10577
(800) 699-3533
www.nutrition21.com (click Our Divisions)

Smart Salt
Mineral Resources International
1990 West and 3300 South
Ogden, UT 84401
(800) 731-7866
www.mineralresourcesint.com

MAGNESIUM TESTING

EXATest
IntraCellular Diagnostics, Inc.
553 Pilgrim Drive, Suite B
Commerce Park
Foster City, CA 94404
(650) 349-5233
Fax (650) 349-9031
E-mail: icd@exatest.com

Ionic Magnesium Testing for Research Purposes:
Drs. Bella and Burton Altura
State University of New York Health Science Center at
Brooklyn
450 Clarkson Avenue
New York, NY 11203
(718) 270-2194 or (718) 270-2205

ORGANIC FOOD

Community Supported Agriculture (CSA)
Become a member in an organic farm CSA in your
community.
(800) 516-7797
www.reeusda.gov/csa.html

HOLISTIC DENTAL ASSOCIATIONS AND BIOLOGICAL DENTISTRY

International Academy of Oral Medicine and Toxicology
8297 Champions Gate Blvd. #193
Champions Gate, FL 33896
(863) 420-6373
http://www.iaomt.org

Holistic Dental Association
P.O. Box 5007
Durango, CO 81301
www.holisticdental.org

HOLISTIC MEDICAL ORGANIZATIONS

The American College for Advancement in Medicine
(ACAM)
23121 Verdugo Drive, Suite 204
Laguna Hills, CA 92653
Fax (949) 455-9679
www.acam.org

American Academy of Environmental Medicine
7701 East Kellogg, Suite 625
Wichita, KS 67207
(316) 684-5500
Fax (316) 684-5709
www.aaem.com

American Academy of Pain Management
13947 Mono Way, #A
Sonora, CA 95370
(209) 533-9744
www.aapainmanage.org

American Holistic Medical Association (AHMA)
6728 McLean Village Drive
McLean, VA 22101-8729
(703) 556-9728
Fax (703) 556-8729
www.holisticmedicine.org

American Association of Preventive Medicine
9912 Georgetown Pike, Suite D-2
P.O. Box 458
Great Falls, VA 22066
(800) 230-AAHF
(703) 759-0662
Fax (703) 759-6711
www.apma.net

The Foundation for the Advancement of Innovative Medicine
(FAIM)
P.O. Box 7016
Albany, NY 12225-0016
(877) 634-3246
Fax (518) 758-7967
www.faim.org

International Society for Orthomolecular Medicine
16 Florence Avenue
Toronto, Ontario, Canada M2N 1E9
(416) 733-2117
Fax (416) 733-2352
www.orthomed.org

American Association of Naturopathic Physicians
8201 Greensboro Drive, Suite 300
McLean, VA 22102
(703) 610-9037
Fax (703) 610-9005
(877) 969-2267
www.naturopathic.org

International and American Associations of Clinical
Nutritionists
16775 Addison Road, Suite 100
Addison, TX 75001
(972) 407-9089
Fax (972) 250-0233
www.iaacn.org

American Holistic Nurses Association
P.O. Box 2130
Flagstaff, AZ 86003-2130
(800) 278-2462
www.ahna.org

REFERENCES

INTRODUCTION

1. Aikawa JK, *Magnesium: Its Biologic Significance*, CRC Press, Boca Raton, FL, 1981.
2. Iannello S, Belfiore F, "Hypomagnesemia. A review of pathophysiological, clinical and therapeutical aspects." *Panminerva Med*, vol. 43, no. 3, pp. 177–209, 2001.
3. Altura BM, "Introduction: importance of Mg in physiology and medicine and the need for ion selective electrodes." *Scand J Clin Lab Invest Suppl*, vol. 217, pp. 5–9, 1994.
4. Institute of Medicine, *Dietary Reference Intake for Calcium, Phosphorus, Magnesium, Vitamin D, and Fluoride*, National Academy Press, Washington DC, 1997.
5. Durlach J, *Magnesium in Clinical Practice*, Libbey, London, 1988.
6. Fehlinger R, "Therapy with magnesium salts in neurological diseases." *Magnes Bull*, vol. 12, pp. 35–42, 1990.
7. Ducroix T, "L'enfant spasmophile—Aspects diagnostiques et thérapeutiques." *Magnes Bull*, vol. 1, pp. 9–15, 1984.

CHAPTER 1: THE CASE FOR MAGNESIUM

1. Altura BM, Altura BT, "Cardiovascular risk factors and magnesium: relationships to atherosclerosis, ischemic heart disease and hypertension." *Magnes Trace Elem*, vol. 92, no. 10, pp. 182–192, 1991.

2. Eisenberg MJ, "Magnesium deficiency and sudden death." *Amer Heart J*, vol. 124, no. 2, pp. 544–549, 1992.

3. Turlapaty PD, Altura BM, "Magnesium deficiency produces spasms of coronary arteries: relationship to etiology of sudden death ischemic heart disease." *Science*, vol. 208, no. 4440, pp. 198–200, 1980.

4. Altura BM, "Sudden-death ischemic heart disease and dietary magnesium intake: is the target site coronary vascular smooth muscle?" *Med Hypotheses*, vol. 5, no. 8, pp. 843–848, 1979.

5. Karppanen H et al., "Minerals, coronary heart disease and sudden coronary death." *Adv Cardiol*, vol. 25, pp. 9–24, 1978.

6. Rogers SA, *Depression Cured at Last*, SK Publishing, Sarasota, FL, 2000.

7. Henrotte JG, "Type A behavior and magnesium metabolism." *Magnesium*, vol. 5, pp. 201–210, 1986.

8. Cernak I et al., "Alterations in magnesium and oxidative status during chronic emotional stress." *Magnes Res*, vol. 13, no. 1, pp. 29–36, 2000.

9. Goldberg B, *Alternative Medicine Guide: Women's Health Series 1*, Future Medicine Publishing, Tiburon, CA, 1998.

10. Aikawa JK, *Magnesium: Its Biologic Significance*, CRC Press, Boca Raton, FL, 1981.

11. Levine BS, Coburn JW, "Magnesium, the mimic/antagonist of calcium." *N Engl J Med*, vol. 310, pp. 1253–1255, 1984.

12. Iseri LT, French JH, "Magnesium: nature's physiologic calcium blocker." *Am Heart J*, vol. 108, pp. 188–193, 1984.

13. Seelig MS, "Cardiovascular reactions to stress intensified by magnesium deficit in consequences of magnesium deficiency on the enhancement of stress reactions; preventive and therapeutic implications: a review." *J Am Coll Nutr*, vol. 13, no. 5, pp. 429–446, 1994.

14. Rodale JR, *Magnesium: The Nutrient That Could Change Your Life*, Rodale Press, Emmaus, PA 1971. Full text available at http://www.mgwater.com/rodtitle.shtml.

15. Hartwig A, "Role of magnesium in genomic stability." *Mutat Research*, vol. 18, no. 475 (1–2), pp. 113–121, 2001.

16. Pfeiffer CC, *Zinc and Other Micro-Nutrients*, Keats, New Canaan, CT, 1978.

17. Walker GM, "Biotechnological implications of the interactions between magnesium and calcium." *Magnes Res*, vol. 12, no. 4, pp. 303–309, 1999.

18. Altura BM, "Sudden-death ischemic heart disease and dietary magnesium intake: is the target site coronary vascular smooth muscle?" *Med Hypotheses*, vol. 8, pp. 843–848, 1979.

19. Eades M, Eades A, *The Protein Power Lifeplan*, Warner Books, New York, 1999.

CHAPTER 2: MAGNESIUM: THE MISSING MINERAL

1. Kant AK, "Consumption of energy-dense, nutrient-poor foods by adult Americans: nutritional and health implications. The third National Health and Nutrition Examination Survey, 1988–1994." *Am J Clin Nutr*, vol. 72, no. 4, pp. 929–936, 2000.

2. Institute of Medicine, *Dietary Reference Intake for Calcium, Phosphorus, Magnesium, Vitamin D, and Fluoride*, National Academy Press, Washington DC, 1997.

3. See www.mgwater.com/leaching.shtml.

4. See www.sunarc.org/JAD97.pdf.

5. Machoy-Mokrzynska, A., "Fluoride_Magnesium Interaction." *Fluoride*, vol. 28, no. 4, pp. 175–177, 1995.

6. "Fluorides, Hydrogen Fluoride, and Fluorine: A Toxicological Profile," U.S. Department of Health and Human Services, Public Health Service, Agency for Toxic Substances and Disease Registry (ATSDR) TP-91/17, page 112, sec. 2.7 (Health Impacts), April 1993.

7. Werbach MR, *Nutritional Influences on Illness*, Thorstons Publishing Group, Wellingborough, Northamptonshire, 1989.

8. Ibid.

9. Graham L, Caesar J, Burger A, "Gastrointestinal absorption and excretion of Mg." *Metabolism*, vol. 9, 1960.

10. Eades M, Eades A, *The Protein Power Lifeplan*, Warner Books, New York, 1999.

11. Ibid.

12. Linderman RD, "Influence of various nutrients and hormones on urinary divalent cation excretion." *Ann NY Acad Sci*, vol. 162, pp. 802–809, 1969.

13. Lemann J et al., "Evidence that glucose ingestion inhibits net renal tubular reabsorption of calcium and magnesium in man." *J Lab Clin Medicine*, vol. 75, pp. 578–585, 1970.

14. Barbagallo M, Dominguez LJ, Resnick LM, "Insulin-mimetic action of vanadate: role of intracellular magnesium." *Hypertension*, vol. 3, pt. 2, pp. 701–704, 2001.

15. *Physicians' Desk Reference*, 56th ed., Medical Economics, Oradell, NJ, 2002.

16. Ibid.

17. Crossen C, *Tainted Truth: The Manipulation of Fact*. Simon & Schuster, New York, 1995.

18. Teo KK et al., "Effects of intravenous magnesium in suspected acute myocardial infarction: overview of randomized trials." *Brit Med J*, vol. 303, pp. 1499–1503, 1991.

19. Teo KK, Yusuf S, "Role of magnesium in reducing mortality in acute myocardial infarction. A review of the evidence." *Drugs*, vol. 46, pp. 347–359, 1993.

20. Altura BM, "Sudden-death ischemic heart disease and dietary magnesium intake: is the target site coronary vascular smooth muscle?" *Med Hypotheses*, vol. 5, no. 8, pp. 843–848, 1979.

21. Altura BM, "Introduction: importance of Mg in physiology and medicine and the need for ion selective electrodes." *Scand J Clin Lab Invest Suppl*, vol. 217, pp. 5–9, 1994.

22. Mauskop A, Fox B, *What Your Doctor May Not Tell You About Migraines*. Warner Books, New York, 2001.

23. Mauskop A et al., "Deficiency in serum ionized magnesium but not total magnesium in patients with migraines. Possible role of ICa2/IMg2 ratio." *Headache*, vol. 33, no. 3, pp. 135–138, 1993.

24. Mauskop A et al., "Intravenous magnesium sulphate relieves migraine attacks in patients with low serum ionized magnesium levels: a pilot study." *Clin Sci (Colch)*, vol. 89, no. 6, pp. 633–636, 1995.

25. Seelig MS, "The requirement of magnesium by the normal adult." *Am J Clin Nutr*, vol. 14, pp. 342–390, 1964.

26. Seelig MS, "Cardiovascular reactions to stress intensified by magnesium deficit in consequences of magnesium deficiency on the enhancement of stress reactions; preventive and therapeutic implications: a review." *J Am Coll Nutr*, vol. 13, no. 5, pp. 429–446, 1994.

27. Durlach J, *Magnesium in Clinical Practice*, Libbey, London, 1988.

28. Durlach J, "Diverse applications of magnesium therapy," in *Handbook of Metal-Ligand Interactions in Biological Fluids—Bioinorganic Medicine*, vol. 2, Marcel Dekker, New York, 1995.

CHAPTER 3: ANXIETY AND DEPRESSION

1. Klerman GL, Weissman MM, "Increasing rates of depression." *JAMA*, vol. 261, no. 15, pp. 2229–2235, 1992.

2. Weissman MM, "Cross-national epidemiology of major depression and bipolar disorder." *JAMA*, vol. 276, no. 4, pp. 293–299, 1996.

3. Murphy JM, "A 40-year perspective on the prevalence of depression: the Stirling County Study." *Arch Gen Psychiatry*, vol. 57, no. 3, pp. 209–215, 2000.

4. Cox RH, Shealy CN, Cady RK, Veehoff D, Burnetti Awell M, Houston R, "Significant magnesium deficiency in depression." *J Neurol Orthop Med Surg*, vol 17, pp. 7–9, 1996.

5. Michiel RR, "Sudden death in a patient on a liquid protein diet." *New Engl J Med*, vol. 298, pp. 1005–1007, 1978.

6. Werbach MR, "Nutritional influences on aggressive behavior." *Journal of Orthomolecular Medicine*, vol. 7, no. 1, 1995.

7. Rogers SA, *Depression Cured at Last*, SK Publishing, Sarasota, FL, 2000.

8. Durlach J, "Diverse applications of magnesium therapy," in *Handbook of Metal-Ligand Interactions in Biological Fluids—Bioinorganic Medicine*, vol. 2, Marcel Dekker, New York, 1995.

9. Penland JG, "Quantitative analysis of EEG effects following experimental marginal magnesium and boron deprivation." *Magnes Res*, vol 8, no. 4, 341–358, 1995.

10. Seelig MS, "Mechanisms of interactions of stress, stress hormones and magnesium in consequences of magnesium deficiency on the enhancement of stress reactions; preventive and therapeutic implications: a review." *J Am Coll Nutr*, vol. 13, no. 5, pp. 429–446, 1994.

11. Cernak I et al., "Alterations in magnesium and oxidative status during chronic emotional stress." *Magnes Res*, vol. 13, pp. 29–36, 2000.

12. Classen HG et al., "Coping with acute stress reaction by plentiful oral magnesium supply." *Magnes Bull*, vol. 17, pp. 1–8, 1995.

13. Mocci F, Canalis P, Tomasi PA, Casu F, Pettinato S, "The effect of noise

on serum and urinary magnesium and catecholamines in humans." *Occup Med (Lond)*, vol. 51, no. 1, pp. 56–61, 2001.

14. Starobrat-Hermelin B, Kozielec T, "The effects of magnesium physiological supplementation on hyperactivity in children with attention deficit hyperactivity disorder (ADHD). Positive response to magnesium oral loading test." *Magnes Res*, vol. 10, no. 2, pp. 149–156, 1997.

15. Olfman, S. *No Child Left Different*, Praeger, Westport, CT, 2006, p. 1

16. Galland L, Buchman Diane D., *Superimmunity for Kids*, Dell, New York, 1988.

17. Rogers SA, *Depression Cured at Last*, SK Publishing, Sarasota, FL, 2000.

CHAPTER 4: MIGRAINES AND PAIN

1. Blaylock RL, *Excitotoxins: The Taste That Kills*, Health Press, Sante Fe, NM, 1997.

2. Ibid.

3. Eades M, Eades A, *The Protein Power Lifeplan*, Warner Books, New York, 1999.

4. Weaver K, "Magnesium and migraine." *Headache*, vol. 30, p. 168, 1990.

5. Mauskop A, Fox B, *What Your Doctor May Not Tell You About Migraines*, Warner Books, New York, 2001.

6. Mauskop A et al., "Deficiency in serum ionized magnesium but not total magnesium in patients with migraines. Possible role of ICa2/IMg2 ratio." *Headache*, vol. 33, no. 3, pp. 135–138, 1993.

7. Ibid.

8. Mauskop A et al., "Intravenous magnesium sulphate relieves migraine attacks in patients with low serum ionized magnesium levels: a pilot study." *Clin Sci (Colch)*, vol. 89, no. 6, pp. 633–636, 1995.

9. Mauskop A, Altura BT et al., "Intravenous magnesium sulfate rapidly alleviates headaches of various types." *Headache*, vol. 36, no. 3, pp. 154–160, 1996.

10. Mauskop A, Altura BM, "Role of magnesium in the pathogenesis and treatment of migraines." *Clin Neurosci*, vol. 83, no. 5, pp. 24–27, 1998.

11. Mauskop A et al., "Intravenous magnesium sulfate relieves cluster

headaches in patients with low serum ionized magnesium levels." *Headache,* vol. 35, no. 10, pp. 597–600, 1995.

12. Mauskop A, Altura BT et al., "Intravenous magnesium sulfate rapidly alleviates headaches of various types." *Headache,* vol. 36, no. 3, pp. 154–160, 1996.

13. Peikert A, Wilimzig C et al., "Prophylaxis of migraine with oral magnesium: results from a prospective, multi-center, placebo-controlled and double-blind randomized study." *Cephalalgia,* vol. 16, no. 4, pp. 257–263, 1996.

14. Crosby V, Wilcock A, Corcoran R, "The safety and efficacy of a single dose (500 mg or 1 g) of intravenous magnesium sulfate in neuropathic pain poorly responsive to strong opioid analgesics in patients with cancer." *J Pain Synmptom Management,* vol. 20, no. 1, pp. 35–39, 2000.

15. See www.ninds.nih.gov/disorders/tourette/detail_tourette.htm.

16. Grimaldi BL, "The central role of magnesium deficiency in Tourette's syndrome: causal relationships between magnesium deficiency, altered biochemical pathways and symptoms relating to Tourette's syndrome and several reported comorbid conditions." *Med Hypotheses,* vol 58, no. 1, pp. 47–60, 2002.

17. Seelig MS, "Athletic stress, performance and magnesium in consequences of magnesium deficiency on the enhancement of stress reactions; preventive and therapeutic implications: a review." *J Am Coll Nutr,* vol. 13, no. 5, pp. 429–446, 1994.

18. Blaylock RL, *Excitotoxins: The Taste That Kills,* Health Press, Santa Fe, NM, 1997.

19. Ibid.

20. Seelig MS, "Athletic stress, performance and magnesium in consequences of magnesium deficiency on the enhancement of stress reactions; preventive and therapeutic implications: a review." *J Am Coll Nutr,* vol. 13, no. 5, pp. 429–446, 1994.

21. Singh RB, "Effect of dietary magnesium supplementation in the prevention of coronary heart disease and sudden cardiac death." *Magnesium Trace Elem,* vol. 9, pp. 143–151, 1990.

22. Stendig-Lindberg G, "Sudden death of athletes: is it due to long-term changes in serum magnesium, lipids and blood sugar?" *J Basic Clin Physiol Pharmacol,* vol. 3, no. 2, pp. 153–164, 1992.

CHAPTER 5: STROKES, HEAD INJURY, AND BRAIN SURGERY

1. Institute of Medicine, *Dietary Reference Intake for Calcium, Phosphorus, Magnesium, Vitamin D, and Fluoride*, National Academy Press, Washington DC, 1997.

2. Blaylock RL, *Excitotoxins: The Taste That Kills*, Health Press, Sante Fe, NM, 1997.

3. Durlach J et al., "Physiopathology of symptomatic and latent forms of central nervous hyperexcitability due to magnesium deficiency: a current general scheme." *Magnes Res*, vol. 13, no. 4, pp. 293–302, 2000.

4. Cernak I et al., "Characterization of plasma magnesium concentration and oxidative stress following graded traumatic brain injury in humans." *J Neurotrauma*, vol. 17, no. 1, pp. 53–68, 2000.

5. Memon ZI et al., "Predictive value of serum ionized but not total magnesium levels in head injuries." *Scand J Clin Lab Invest*, vol. 55, no. 8, pp. 671–677, 1995.

6. Heath DL, Vink R, "Brain free magnesium concentration is predictive of motor outcome following traumatic axonal brain injury in rats." *Magnes Res*, vol. 12, no. 4, pp. 269–277, 1999.

7. Blaylock RL, *Excitotoxins: The Taste That Kills*, Health Press, Sante Fe, NM, 1997.

8. Marcus JC et al., "Serum ionized magnesium in post-traumatic headaches." *J Pediatr*, vol. 139, no. 3, pp. 459–462, 2001.

9. Altura BM, Altura BT, "Association of alcohol in brain injury, headaches, and stroke with brain-tissue and serum levels of ionized magnesium: a review of recent findings and mechanisms of action." *Alcohol*, vol. 19, no. 2, pp. 119–130, 1999.

10. Altura BM et al., "Alcohol-induced spasms of cerebral blood vessels: relation to cerebrovascular accidents and sudden death." *Science*, vol. 220, no. 4594, pp. 331–333, 1983.

11. Zhang A et al., "Chronic treatment of cultured cerebral vascular smooth cells with low concentration of ethanol elevates intracellular calcium and potentiates prostanoid-induced rises in [Ca2+]i: relation to etiology of alcohol-induced stroke." *Alcohol*, vol. 14, no. 4, pp. 367–371, 1997.

12. Altura BM, Altura BT, "Association of alcohol in brain injury,

headaches, and stroke with brain-tissue and serum levels of ionized magnesium: a review of recent findings and mechanisms of action." *Alcohol*, vol. 19, no. 2, pp. 119–130, 1999.

13. Abbot L et al., "Magnesium deficiency in alcoholism: possible contribution to osteoporosis and cardiovascular disease in alcoholics." *Alcohol Clin Exp Res*, vol. 19, pp. 1076–1082, 1994.

14. Altura BM, Altura BT, "Association of alcohol in brain injury, headaches, and stroke with brain-tissue and serum levels of ionized magnesium: a review of recent findings and mechanisms of action." *Alcohol*, vol. 19, no. 2, pp. 119–130, 1999.

15. Altura BM et al., "Extracellular magnesium regulates nuclear and perinuclear free ionized calcium in cerebral vascular smooth muscle cells: possible relation to alcohol and central nervous system injury." *Alcohol*, vol. 23, no. 2, pp. 83–90, 2001.

16. Ema M et al., "Alcohol-induced vascular damage of brain is ameliorated by administration of magnesium." *Alcohol*, vol. 15, no. 2, pp. 95–103, 1998.

17. Yang CY, "Calcium and magnesium in drinking water and risk of death from cerebrovascular disease." *Stroke*, vol. 18, no. 8, pp. 411–414, 1998.

18. Altura BM, Altura BT, "Association of alcohol in brain injury, headaches, and stroke with brain-tissue and serum levels of ionized magnesium: a review of recent findings and mechanisms of action." *Alcohol*, vol. 19, no. 2, pp. 119–130, 1999.

19. Li W et al., "Antioxidants prevent depletion of [Mg2+]i induced by alcohol in cultured canine cerebral vascular smooth muscle cells: possible relationship to alcohol-induced stroke." *Brain Res Bull*, vol. 55, no. 4, pp. 475–478, 2001.

20. See http://www.nfam.org/2004yearendnewsletter_stroke.html.

21. Horn B, "Magnesium and the cardiovascular system." *Magnesium*, vol. 6, pp. 109–111, 1987.

22. Schulz-Stubner S et al., "Magnesium as part of balanced general anaesthesia with propofol, remifentanil and mivacurium: a double-blind, randomized prospective study in 50 patients." *Eur J Anaesthesiol*, vol. 18, no. 11, pp. 723–729, 2001.

23. Altura BT, Altura BM, "Withdrawal of magnesium causes vasospasm while elevated magnesium produces relaxation of tone

in cerebral arteries." *Neurosci Lett*, vol. 20, no. 3, pp. 323–327, 1980.

24. Altura BT, Altura BM, "Interactions of Mg and K on cerebral vessels—aspects in view of stroke. Review of present status and new findings." *Magnesium*, vol. 3, nos. 4–6, pp. 195–211, 1984.

25. Li W et al., "Antioxidants prevent elevation in [Ca(2+)](i) induced by low extracellular magnesium in cultured canine cerebral vascular smooth muscle cells: possible relationship to Mg(2+) deficiency-induced vasospasm and stroke." *Brain Res Bull*, vol. 52, no. 2, pp. 151–154, 2000.

26. Blaylock RL, *Excitotoxins: The Taste That Kills*, Health Press, Sante Fe, NM, 1997, p. 181.

27. Ibid.

28. Altura BT et al., "Low levels of serum ionized magnesium are found in patients early after stroke which result in rapid elevation in cytosolic free calcium and spasm in cerebral vascular muscle cells." *Neurosci Lett*, vol. 230, no. 1, pp. 37–40, 1997.

29. Galland L, Buchman Diane D., *Superimmunity for Kids*, Dell, New York, 1988.

CHAPTER 6: CHOLESTEROL AND HYPERTENSION

1. Goldberg B, *Heart Disease*, Future Medicine Publishing, Tiburon, CA, 1998.

2. Altura BT et al., "Magnesium dietary intake modulates blood lipid levels and artherogenesis." *Proc Natl Acad Sci*, vol. 87, no. 5, pp. 1840–1844, 1990.

3. Singh RB et al., "Does dietary magnesium modulate blood lipids?" *Biol Trace Elem Res*, vol. 30, pp. 50–64, 1991.

4. Corica F et al., "Effects of oral magnesium supplementation on plasma lipid concentrations in patients with non-insulin-dependent diabetes mellitus." *Magnesium Res*, vol. 7, pp. 43–46, 1994.

5. Durlach J, "Commentary on recent epidemiological and clinical advances." *Magnesium Research*, vol. 9, no. 2, pp. 139–141, 1996.

6. Fallon S, Enig M, *Nourishing Traditions*, Locomotion Press, Baltimore, MD, 1995.

7. Gao M et al., "Cardiovascular risk factors emerging in Chinese populations undergoing urbanization." *Hypertens Res*, vol. 22, pp. 209–215, 1999.

8. Marier JR, "Magnesium content of the food supply in the modern-day world." *Magnesium*, vol. 5, pp. 1–8, 1986.

9. Liu L et al., "Comparative studies of diet-related factors and blood pressure among Chinese and Japanese: results from the China-Japan Cooperative Research of the WHO-CARDIAC Study. Cardiovascular disease and alimentary comparison." *Hypertens Res*, vol. 23, pp. 413–420, 2000.

10. Friedland GW, Friedman M, *Medicine's 10 Greatest Discoveries*, Yale University Press, New Haven, CT, 1998.

11. Ford R, *Stale Food vs. Fresh Food: The Cause and Cure of Choked Arteries and Related Problems*, Magnolia Laboratories, Pascagoula, MS, 1969.

12. Erasmus U, *Fats That Heal, Fats That Kill*, Alive Books, Burnaby, BC, 1993, p. 64.

13. Rosanoff A, Seelig MS, "Comparison of mechanism and functional effects of magnesium and statin pharmaceuticals." *J Am Coll Nutr*, vol. 23, no. 5, pp. 501S–505S, 2004.

14. McCully KS, "Homocysteine, folate, vitamin B_6, and cardiovascular disease." *JAMA*, vol. 279, no. 5, pp. 392–393, 1998.

15. McCully KS, "Vascular pathology of homocysteinemia: implications for the pathogenesis of arteriosclerosis." *Am J Pathol*, vol. 56, no. 1, pp. 111–128, 1969.

16. Eikelboom JW et al., "Preventive cardiology and therapeutics program." *Ann Intern Med*, vol. 131, no. 5, pp. 363–375, 1999.

17. Boushey CJ et al., "A quantitative assessment of plasma homocysteine as a risk factor for vascular disease. Probable benefits of increasing folic acid intakes." *JAMA*, vol. 274, no. 13, pp. 1049–1057, 1995.

18. Confalonieri M et al., "Heterozygosity for homocysteinuria: a detectable and reversible risk factor for pulmonary thromboembolism." *Monaldi Arch Chest Disease*, vol. 50, no. 2, pp. 114–115, 1995.

19. Altura B, Altura B, "Magnesium: the forgotten mineral in cardiovascular health and disease." A Gem Lecture at SUNY Downstate. *Alumni Today*, pp. 11–22, spring 2001.

20. Li W et al., "Extracellular magnesium regulates effects of vitamin B_6, B_{12} and folate on homocysteinemia-induced depletion of intracellular free magnesium ions in canine cerebral vascular smooth muscle cells: possible relationship to [Ca2+]i, atherogenesis and stroke." *Neurosci Lett*, vol. 274, no. 2, pp. 83–86, 1999.

21. Shamsuddin AM, "Inositol phosphates have novel anti-cancer function." *Journal of Nutrition*, vol. 125 (suppl.), pp. 725S–732S, Review 1995.

22. Rowley KG et al., "Improvements in circulating cholesterol, antioxidants, and homocysteine after dietary intervention in an Australian Aboriginal community." *Am J Clin Nutr*, vol. 74, no. 4, pp. 442–448, 2001.

23. Tice JA et al., "Cost-effectiveness of vitamin therapy to lower plasma homocysteine levels for the prevention of coronary heart disease: effect of grain fortification and beyond." *JAMA*, vol. 286, no. 8, pp. 936–943, 2001.

24. Vollset SE et al., "Plasma total homocysteine and cardiovascular and noncardiovascular mortality: the Hordaland Homocysteine Study." *Am J Clin Nutr*, vol. 74, no. 1, pp. 130–136, 2001.

25. Batmanghelidj F, *Your Body's Many Cries for Water*, Global Health Solutions, Falls Church, VA, 1997.

26. Altura BM et al., "Hypomagnesemia and vasoconstriction: possible relationship to etiology of sudden death ischemic heart disease and hypertensive vascular diseases." *Artery*, vol. 9, no. 3, pp. 212–231, 1981.

27. Mindell E, *Prescription Alternatives*, Keats Publishing, Los Angeles, 1999.

28. Pierce JB, *Heart Healthy Magnesium: Your Nutritional Key to Cardiovascular Wellness*, Avery Publishing Group, New York, 1994.

29. Millane T, Camm A, *Medical Sciences Bulletin*, Pharmaceutical Information Associates, May 1994.

30. Kisters K et al., "Hypomagnesaemia, borderline hypertension and hyperlipidaemia." *Magnesium Bull*, vol. 21, pp. 31–34, 1999.

31. Altura BM, Altura BT et al., "Magnesium deficiency and hypertension: correlation between magnesium-deficient diets and microcirculatory changes in situ." *Science*, vol. 223, no. 4642, pp. 1315–1317, 1984.

32. Resnick LM et al., "Factors affecting blood pressure responses to diet: the Vanguard study." *Am J Hypertens*, vol. 13, no. 9, pp. 956–965, 2000.

33. Altura BM, Altura BT, "Interactions of Mg and K on blood vessels—aspects in view of hypertension. Review of present status and new findings." *Magnesium*, vol. 3, nos. 4–6, pp. 175–194, 1984.

CHAPTER 7: MAGNESIUM AND HEART DISEASE

1. Lukaski HC, Nielsen FH. "Dietary magnesium depletion affects metabolic responses during submaximal exercise in postmenopausal women." *J Nutr*, vol. 132, no. 5, pp. 930–935, 2002.

2. Goldberg B, *Heart Disease*, Future Medicine Publishing, Tiburon, CA, 1998.

3. Sei M et al., "Nutritional epidemiological study on mineral intake and mortality from cardiovascular disease." *Tokushima J Exp Med*, vol. 40, nos. 3–4, pp. 199–207, 1993.

4. Zwillinger L, "Effect of magnesium on the heart." *Klin Wochenschr*, vol. 14, pp. 1429–1433, 1935.

5. Tom Miller, personal communication, March 2001.

6. Singh RB, "Magnesium status and risk of coronary artery disease in rural and urban populations with variable magnesium consumption." *Magnes Res*, vol. 10, no. 3, pp. 205–213, 1997.

7. Liao F, Folsom AR, "Is low magnesium concentration a risk factor for coronary heart disease? The atherosclerosis risk in communities (ARIC) study." *Am Heart J*, vol. 136, no. 3, pp. 480–490, 1998.

8. Ford, Earl S. "Serum magnesium and ischemic heart disease: findings from a national sample of US adults." *International Journal of Epidemiology*, vol. 28, pp. 645–651, 1999.

9. Seelig MS, Heggtveit HA, "Magnesium interrelationships in ischemic heart disease: a review." *Am J Clin Nutr*, vol. 27, no. 1, pp. 59–79, 1974.

10. Sherer Y, Bitzur R, Cohen H, Shaish A, Varon D, Shoenfeld Y, Harats D, "Mechanisms of action of the anti-atherogenic effect of magnesium: lessons from a mouse model." *Magnes Res*, vol. 14, no. 3, pp. 173–179, 2001.

11. Morrill GA, Gupta RK, Kostellow AB, Ma GY, Zhang A, Altura BT, Altura BM, "Mg2 modulates membrane sphingolipid and lipid second

messenger levels in vascular smooth muscle cells." *FEBS Lett*, vol. 440, nos. 1–2, pp. 167–171, 1998.

12. Yang ZW, Gebrewold A et al., "Mg++-induced endothelial-dependent relaxation of blood vessels and blood pressure lowering: role of NO." *Am J Physiol Regul Integr Comp Physiol*, vol. 278, pp. R628–639, 2000.

13. Kang DH, Park SK, Lee IK, Johnson RJ, "Uric acid–induced C-reactive protein expression: implication on cell proliferation and nitric oxide production of human vascular cells." *J Am Soc Nephrol*, vol. 16, no. 12, pp. 3553–3562, 2005.

14. *Physicians' Desk Reference*, 56th ed., Medical Economics, Oradell, NJ, 2002.

15. Pierce JB, *Heart Healthy Magnesium: Your Nutritional Key to Cardiovascular Wellness*, Avery Publishing Group, New York, 1994.

16. Shechter M et al., "Beneficial antithrombotic effects of the association of pharmacological oral magnesium therapy with aspirin in coronary heart disease patients." *Magnes Research*, vol. 13, no. 4, pp. 275–284, 2000.

17. Zwillinger L, "Effect of magnesium on the heart." *Klin Wochenschr*, vol. 14, pp. 1429–1433, 1935.

18. Boyd LJ et al., "Magnesium sulfate in paroxysmal tachycardia." *Am J Med Sci*, vol. 206, pp. 43–48, 1943.

19. Teo KK et al., "Effects of intravenous magnesium in suspected acute myocardial infarction: overview of randomized trials." *Brit Med J*, vol. 303, pp. 1499–1503, 1991.

20. Teo KK, Yusuf S, "Role of magnesium in reducing mortality in acute myocardial infarction. A review of the evidence." *Drugs*, vol. 46, pp. 347–359, 1993.

21. Woods KL et al., "Intravenous magnesium sulfate in suspected acute myocardial infarction: results of the second Leicester Intravenous Magnesium Intervention Trial (LIMIT-2)." *Lancet*, vol. 339, pp. 1553–1558, 1992.

22. Woods KL, Fletcher S, "Long-term outcome after intravenous magnesium sulphate in suspected acute myocardial infarction: the second Leicester Intravenous Magnesium Intervention Trial (LIMIT-2)." *Lancet*, vol. 343, pp. 816–819, 1994.

23. Ravn HB, "Pharmacological effects of magnesium on arterial

thrombosis—mechanisms of action?" *Magnes Research*, vol. 12, no. 3, pp. 191–199, 1999.

24. Young IS et al., "Magnesium status and digoxin toxicity." *Br J Clin Pharmacol*, vol. 32, no. 6, pp. 717–721, 1991.

25. Lewis R et al., "Magnesium deficiency may be an important determinant of ventricular ectopy in digitalised patients with chronic atrial fibrillation." *Br J Clin Pharmacol*, vol. 31, no. 2, pp. 200–203, 1991.

26. ISIS-4 (Fourth International Study of Infarct Survival) Collaborative Group, "ISIS-4: a randomised factorial trial assessing early oral captopril, oral mononitrate, and intravenous magnesium sulphate in 58,050 patients with suspected acute myocardial infarction." *Lancet*, vol. 345, pp. 669–685, 1995.

27. Seelig MS, "Cardiovascular reactions to stress intensified by magnesium deficit in consequences of magnesium deficiency on the enhancement of stress reactions; preventive and therapeutic implications: a review." *J Am Coll Nutr*, vol. 13, no. 5, pp. 429–446, 1994.

28. Shechter M, Shechter A, "Magnesium and myocardial infarction." *Clin Calcium*, vol. 15, no. 11, pp. 111–115, 2005.

29. Shecter M, Bairey Merz CN, Stuehlinger HG, Slany J, Pachinger O, Rabinowitz B, "Effects of oral magnesium therapy on exercise tolerance, exercise-induced chest pain, and quality of life in patients with coronary artery disease." *Am J Cardiol*, vol. 91, no. 5, pp. 517–521, 2003.

30. Shecter M, "Does magnesium have a role in the treatment of patients with coronary artery disease?" *Am J Cardiovasc Drugs*, vol. 3, no. 4, pp. 231–239, 2003.

31. Shechter M, Hod H, Rabinowitz B, Boyko V, Chouraqui P, "Long-term outcome of intravenous magnesium therapy in thrombolysis-ineligible acute myocardial infarction patients." *Cardiology*, vol. 99, no. 4, pp. 205–210, 2003.

32. Shechter M, Sharir M, Labrador MJ, Forrester J, Silver B, Bairey Merz CN, "Oral magnesium therapy improves endothelial function in patients with coronary artery disease." *Circulation*, vol. 102, no. 19, pp. 2353–2358, 2000.

33. Shechter M, Merz CN, Rude RK, Paul Labrador MJ, Meisel SR, Shah PK, Kaul S, "Low intracellular magnesium levels promote platelet-

dependent thrombosis in patients with coronary artery disease." *Am Heart J*, vol. 140, no. 2, pp. 212–218, 2000.

34. Shechter M et al., "Magnesium therapy in acute myocardial infarction when patients are not candidates for thrombolytic therapy." *AM J Cardiology*, vol. 75, pp. 321–323, 1995.

35. Pierce JB, *Heart Healthy Magnesium: Your Nutritional Key to Cardiovascular Wellness*, Avery Publishing Group, New York, 1994.

36. Iseri LT, "Magnesium and cardiac arrhythmias." *Magnesium*, vol. 5, nos. 3–4, pp. 111–126, 1986.

37. Iseri LT, Allen BJ, "Magnesium therapy of cardiac arrhythmias in critical-care medicine." *Magnesium*, vol. 8, pp. 299–306, 1989.

38. Perticone F et al., "Antiarrhythmic short-term protective magnesium treatment in ischemic dilated cardiomyopathy." *J Am Coll Nutr*, vol. 5, no. 3, pp. 492–499, 1990.

39. Pierce JB, *Heart Healthy Magnesium: Your Nutritional Key to Cardiovascular Wellness*, Avery Publishing Group, New York, 1994.

40. Boyd LJ et al., "Magnesium sulfate in paroxysmal tachycardia." *Am J Med Sci*, vol. 206, pp. 43–48, 1943.

41. Parikka HJ, Toivonen LK, "Acute effects of intravenous magnesium on ventricular refractoriness and monophasic action potential duration in humans." *Scand Cardiovasc J*, vol. 33, no. 5, pp. 300–305, 1999.

42. Thiele R, Protze F, Winnefeld K, Pfeifer R, Pleissner J, Gassel M, "Effect of intravenous magnesium on ventricular tachyarrhythmias associated with acute myocardial infarction." *Magnes Res*, vol. 13, no. 2, pp. 111–112, 2000.

43. Ceremuzynski L et al., "Hypomagnesaemia in heart failure with ventricular arrhythmias. Beneficial effects of magnesium supplementation." *J Intern Med*, vol. 247, pp. 78–86, 2000.

44. Dyckner T et al., "Magnesium deficiency in congestive heart failure." *Acta Pharmacol Toxicol Copenh*, vol. 54, suppl. 1, pp. 119–123, 1984.

45. England MR et al., "Magnesium administration and dysrhythmias after cardiac surgery." *JAMA*, vol. 268, pp. 2395–2402, 1992.

46. Caspi J et al., "Effects of magnesium on myocardial function after coronary artery bypass grafting." *Ann Thorac Surg*, vol. 59, pp. 942–947, 1995.

47. Toraman F, Karabulut EH, Alhan HC, Dagdelen S, Tarcan S, "Magnesium infusion dramatically decreases the incidence of atrial fibrillation after coronary artery bypass grafting." *Ann Thorac Surg,* vol. 72, no. 4, pp. 1256–1261, 2001.

48. Seelig MS, "Review and hypothesis: might patients with the chronic fatigue syndrome have latent tetany of magnesium deficiency." *J Chron Fatigue Syndr,* vol. 4, pp. 77–108, 1998.

49. Lichodziejewsa B et al., "Clinical symptoms of mitral valve prolapse are related to hypomagnesemia and attenuated by magnesium supplementation." *Amer J Cardiology,* vol. 79, pp. 768–772, 1997.

CHAPTER 8: OBESITY, SYNDROME X, AND DIABETES

1. Singh RB, "Association of low plasma concentrations of antioxidant vitamins, magnesium and zinc with high body fat per cent in Indian men." *Magnes Res,* vol. 11, no. 1, pp. 3–10, 1998.

2. Ma J et al., "Associations of serum and dietary magnesium with cardiovascular disease, hypertension, diabetes, insulin, and carotid arterial wall thickness; the ARIC study, Artherosclerosis Risk in Communities Study." *J Clin Epidemiol,* vol. 48, pp. 927–940, 1995.

3. Humphries S et al., "Low dietary magnesium is associated with insulin resistance in a sample of young, non-diabetic Black Americans." *Am J Hypertens,* vol. 12, no. 8, pt. 1, pp. 747–756, 1999.

4. Alzaid AA et al., "Effects of insulin on plasma magnesium in noninsulindependent diabetes mellitus: evidence for insulin resistance." *J Clin Endocrinol Metab,* vol. 80, no. 4, pp. 1376–1381, 1995.

5. Barbagallo M et al., "Altered cellular magnesium responsiveness to hyperglycemia in hypertensive subjects." *Hypertension,* vol. 38, no. 3, pt. 2, pp. 612–615, 2001.

6. Dominguez LJ et al., "Magnesium responsiveness to insulin and insulin-like growth factor I in erythrocytes from normotensive and hypertensive subjects." *J Clin Endocrinol Metab,* vol. 83, no. 12, pp. 4402–4407, 1998.

7. Resnick LM, "Cellular ions in hypertension, insulin resistance, obesity, and diabetes: a unifying theme." *J Am Soc Nephrol,* vol. 3 (4 suppl.), pp. 578–585, 1992.

8. Karppanen H, Neuvonen PJ, "Ischaemic heart-disease and soil magnesium in Finland: water hardness and magnesium in heart muscle." *The Lancet*, Dec. 15, 1973.

9. Resnick LM, "Ionic basis of hypertension, insulin resistance, vascular disease, and related disorders. The mechanism of Syndrome X." *Am J Hypertens*, vol. 6, no. 5, pt. 1, pp. 413–417, 1993.

10. Resnick LM, "The cellular ionic basis of hypertension and allied clinical conditions." *Prog Cardiovasc Dis*, vol. 42, pp. 1–22, 1999.

11. Resnick LM et al., "Hypertension and peripheral insulin resistance. Possible mediating role of intracellular free magnesium." *Am J Hypertens*, vol. 3, no. 5, pt. 1, pp. 373–379, 1990.

12. He K, Liu K, Daviglus ML, Morris SJ, Loria CM, Van Horn L, Jacobs DR, Savage PJ, "Magnesium intake and incidence of metabolic syndrome among young adults." *Circulation*, vol. 113, no. 13, pp. 1675–1682, 2006.

13. Paolisso G et al., "Low fasting and insulin-mediated intracellular magnesium accumulation in hypertensive patients with left ventricular hypertrophy; role of insulin resistance." *Hypertens*, vol. 9, pp. 199–203, 1995.

14. Nadler JL et al., "Magnesium deficiency produces insulin resistance and increased thromboxane synthesis." *Hypertension*, vol. 21, no. 6, pt. 2, pp. 1024–1029, 1993.

15. Bardicef M et al., "Extracellular and intracellular magnesium depletion in pregnancy and gestational diabetes." *Am J Obstet Gynecol*, vol. 172, no. 3, pp. 1009–1013, 1995.

16. Resnick LM et al., "Intracellular and extracellular magnesium depletion in type 2 (non-insulin-dependent) diabetes mellitus." *Diabetologia*, vol. 36, no. 8, pp. 767–770, 1993.

17. Kao WH et al., "Serum and dietary magnesium and the risk for type 2 diabetes mellitus: the Atherosclerosis Risk in Communities Study." *Arch Intern Med*, vol. 159, no. 18, pp. 2151–2159, 1999.

18. Lima M de L, "The effect of magnesium supplementation in increasing doses on the control of type 2 diabetes." *Diabetes Care*, vol. 83, no. 5, pp. 682–686, 1998.

19. Paolisso G, Barbagallo M, "Hypertension, diabetes mellitus, and insulin resistance: the role of intracellular magnesium." *Am J Hypertens*, vol. 10, no. 3, pp. 346–355, 1997.

20. Merz CN et al., "Oral magnesium supplementation inhibits platelet-dependent thrombosis in patients with coronary artery disease." *Am J Cardiol*, vol. 84, pp. 152–156, 1999.

21. Lima M de L, "The effect of magnesium supplementation in increasing doses on the control of type 2 diabetes." *Diabetes Care*, vol. 83, no. 5, pp. 682–686, 1998.

22. Engelen W, Bouten A, De Leeuw I, De Block C, "Are low magnesium levels in type 1 diabetes associated with electromyographical signs of polyneuropathy?" *Magnes Res*, vol. 13, no. 3, pp. 197–203, 2000.

23. Djurhuus MS et al., "Effect of moderate improvement in metabolic control on magnesium and lipid concentrations in patients with type 1 diabetes." *Diabetes Care*, vol. 22, no. 4, pp. 546–554, 1999.

24. Squires S, "The amazing statistics and dangers of soda pop." *Washington Post*, February 27, 2001, p. HE10.

25. Ludwig DS et al., "Relation between consumption of sugar-sweetened drinks and childhood obesity: a prospective, observational analysis." *Lancet*, vol. 357, no. 9255, pp. 505–508, 2001.

26. Bernstein J et al., "Depression of lymphocyte transformation following oral glucose ingestion." *Am J Clin Nutr*, vol. 30, p. 613, 1977.

27. Sanchez A et al., "Role of sugars in human neutrophilic phagocytosis." *Am J Clin Nutr*, vol. 26, no. 11, pp. 1180–1184, 1973.

28. Kijak E et al., "Relationship of blood sugar level and leukocytic phagocytosis." *S Calif State Dent Assoc J*, vol. 32, no. 9, 1964.

29. Lima M de L, "The effect of magnesium supplementation in increasing doses on the control of type 2 diabetes." *Diabetes Care*, vol. 83, no. 5, pp. 682–686, 1998.

30. Yang CY et al., "Magnesium in drinking water and the risk of death from diabetes mellitus." *Magnes Res*, vol. 12, no. 2, pp. 131–137, 1999.

31. Zhao HX et al., "Drinking water composition and childhood-onset type 1 diabetes mellitus in Devon and Cornwall, England." *Diabet Med*, vol. 18, no. 9, pp. 709–717, 2001.

32. Howard JMH, "Magnesium deficiency in peripheral vascular disease." *J Nutritional Med*, vol. 1, p. 39, 1990.

33. Roberts HJ, *Aspartame Disease: An Ignored Epidemic*, Sunshine Sentinel Press, West Palm Beach, FL, 2001.

CHAPTER 9: PMS, DYSMENORRHEA, AND POLYCYSTIC OVARIAN SYNDROME

1. Werbach M, "Premenstrual syndrome: magnesium." *Townsend Letter for Doctors*, June 1995, p. 26.

2. Sherwood RA et al., "Magnesium and the premenstrual syndrome." *Ann Clin Biochem*, vol. 23, no. 6, pp. 667–670, 1986.

3. Posaci et al., "Plasma copper, zinc and magnesium levels in patients with premenstrual tension syndrome." *ACTA Obstetrics and Gynecology Scand*, vol. 73, no. 6, pp. 452–455, 1994.

4. Facchinetti F et al., "Oral magnesium successfully relieves premenstrual mood changes." *Obstetrics and Gynecology (USA)*, vol. 78, no. 2, pp. 177–181, 1991.

5. Somer E, *The Essential Guide to Vitamins and Minerals*, HarperCollins, New York, 1995.

6. Murray M, *Encyclopedia of Natural Medicine*, 2nd ed., Prima Publishing, Rocklin, CA, 1998.

7. Muneyvirci-Delale O et al., "Sex steroid hormones modulate serum ionized magnesium and calcium levels throughout the menstrual cycle in women." *Fertil Steril*, vol. 69, no. 5, pp. 58–62, 1998.

8. Li W et al., "Sex steroid hormones exert biphasic effects on cytosolic magnesium ions in cerebral vascular smooth muscle cells: possible relationships to migraine frequency in premenstrual syndromes and stroke incidence." *Brain Res Bull*, vol. 54, no. 1, pp. 83–89, 2001.

9. Marz R, *Medical Nutrition from Marz*, 2nd ed., Omni Press, Portland, OR, 1997.

10. Benassi L et al., "Effectiveness of magnesium picolate in the prophylactic treatment of primary dysmenorrhea." *Clin Exp Obstet Gynecol*, vol. 19, no. 3, pp. 176–179, 1992.

11. Fontana-Klaiber H, Hogg B, "Therapeutic effects of magnesium in dysmenorrhea." *Schweiz Rundsch Med Prax*, vol. 79, no. 16, pp. 491–494, 1990.

12. Seifert B et al., "Magnesium—a new therapeutic alternative in primary dysmenorrhea." *Zentralbl Gynakol*, vol. 111, no. 11, pp. 755–760, 1989.

13. Muneyvirci-Delale O et al., "Divalent cations in women with PCOS: implications for cardiovascular disease." *Gynecol Endocrinol*, vol. 15, no. 3, pp. 198–201, 2001.

CHAPTER 10: INFERTILITY, PREGNANCY, PREECLAMPSIA, AND CEREBRAL PALSY

1. Goldberg B, *Alternative Medicine Guide: Women's Health Series 1*, Future Medicine Publishing, Tiburon, CA, 1998.

2. Franz KB, "Magnesium intake during pregnancy." *Magnesium*, vol. 6, pp. 18–27, 1987.

3. Edorh AP, Tachev K, Hadou T, Gbeassor M, Sanni A, Creppy EE, Le Faou A, Rihn BH, "Magnesium content in seminal fluid as an indicator of chronic prostatitis." *Cell Mol Biol*, vol. 49, pp. 419–423, 2003.

4. Conradt A, Weidinger AH, "The central position of magnesium in the management of fetal hypotrophy—a contribution to the pathomechanism of utero-placental insufficiency, prematurity and poor intrauterine fetal growth as well as pre-eclampsia." *Magnesium Bull*, vol. 4, pp. 103–124, 1982.

5. Handwerker SM et al., "Ionized serum magnesium levels in umbilical cord blood of normal pregnant women at delivery: relationship to calcium, demographics, and birthweight." *Am J Perinatol*, vol. 10, no. 5, pp. 392–397, 1993.

6. Handwerker SM, Altura BT, Altura BM, "Serum ionized magnesium and other electrolytes in the antenatal period of human pregnancy." *J Am Coll Nutr*, vol. 15, no. 1, pp. 36–43, 1996.

7. Almonte RA et al., "Gestational magnesium deficiency is deleterious to fetal outcome." *Biol Neonate*, vol. 76, no. 1, pp. 26–32, 1999.

8. Seelig MS, "Toxemias of pregnancy, postpartum cardiomyopathy and SIDS in consequences of magnesium deficiency on the enhancement of stress reactions; preventive and therapeutic implications: a review." *J Am Coll Nutr*, vol. 13, no. 5, pp. 429–446, 1994.

9. Lazard EM, "A preliminary report on the intravenous use of magnesium sulphate in puerperal eclampsia." *Am J Obst Gynec*, vol. 9, pp. 178–188, 1925.

10. Seelig MS, *Magnesium Deficiency in the Pathogenesis of Disease: Early Roots of Cardiovascular, Skeletal, and Renal Abnormalities*, Plenum, New York, 1980.

11. Seelig MS, "Prenatal and neonatal mineral deficiencies: magnesium, zinc and chromium." In *Clinical Disorders in Pediatric Nutrition*, Marcel Dekker, New York, pp. 167–196, 1982.

12. Seelig MS, "Magnesium in pregnancy: special needs for the adolescent mother." *J Am Coll Nutr,* vol. 10, p. 566, 1991.

13. Caddell JL, "Magnesium deficiency promotes muscle weakness, contributing to the risk of sudden infant death (SIDS) in infants sleeping prone." *Magnes Res,* vol. 14, nos. 1–2, pp. 39–50, 2001.

14. Caddell JL, "A triple-risk model for the sudden infant death syndrome (SIDS) and the apparent life-threatening episode (ALTE): the stressed magnesium deficient weanling rat." *Magnes Res,* vol. 14, no. 3, pp. 227–238, 2001.

15. Durlach J et al., "Magnesium and thermoregulation. I. Newborn and infant. Is sudden infant death syndrome a magnesium-dependent disease of the transition from chemical to physical thermoregulation." *Magnes Res,* vol. 4, pp. 137–152, 1991.

16. Nelson KB et al., "Can magnesium sulfate reduce the risk of cerebral palsy in very low birth weight infants?" *Pediatrics,* vol. 95, no. 2, 1995.

17. Schendel D et al., "Prenatal magnesium sulfate exposure and the risk for cerebral palsy or mental retardation among very low birthweight children aged 3–5 years." *JAMA,* vol. 276, pp. 1805–1810, 1996.

18. Dedhia HV, Banks DE, "Pulmonary response to hyperoxia: effects of magnesium." *Environ Health Perspect,* vol. 102, suppl. 10, pp. 101–105, 1994.

19. Oorschot DE, "Cerebral palsy and experimental hypoxia-induced perinatal brain injury: is magnesium protective?" *Magnes Res,* vol. 13, no. 4, pp. 265–273, 2000.

20. Bara M, Guiet-Bara A, "Magnesium regulation of Ca2+ channels in smooth muscle and endothelial cells of human allantochorial placental vessels." *Magnes Research,* vol. 14, nos. 1–2, pp. 11–18, 2001.

CHAPTER 11: OSTEOPOROSIS AND KIDNEY STONES

1. Brown S, *Better Bones, Better Body,* Keats Publishing, New Canaan, CT, 1996.

2. Thomas AJ et al., "Ca, Mg and P status of elderly inpatients: dietary intake, metabolic balance studies and biochemical status." *Br. J. Nutr,* vol. 62, pp. 211–219, 1989.

3. Bunker VW, "Osteoporosis in the elderly." *Br J Biomed Sci,* vol. 51, no. 3, pp. 228–240, 1994.

4. The National Institutes of Health Osteoporosis Prevention, Diagnosis, and Therapy Consensus Statement, Mar. 2000.

5. Rude RK, "Magnesium deficiency-induced osteoporosis in the rat: uncoupling of bone formation and bone resorption." *Magnes Research,* vol. 12, no. 4, pp. 257–267, 1999.

6. Rude RK et al., "Magnesium deficiency induces bone loss in the rat." *Miner Electrolyte Metab,* vol. 24, no. 5, pp. 314–320, 1998.

7. Brodowski J, "Levels of ionized magnesium in women with various stages of postmenopausal osteoporosis progression evaluated on the basis of densitometric examinations." *Przegl Lek,* vol. 57, no. 12, pp. 714–716, 2000.

8. Sojka JE, Weaver CM, "Magnesium supplementation and osteoporosis," *Nutrition Reviews,* vol. 53, p. 71, 1995.

9. Goldberg B, *Alternative Medicine Guide: Women's Health Series 2,* Future Medicine Publishing, Tiburon, CA, 1998.

10. Dreosti IE, "Magnesium status and health." *Nutrition Reviews,* vol. 53, no. 9, pp. 523–527, 1995.

11. Abraham GE, Grewal HA, "Total dietary program emphasizing magnesium instead of calcium: effect on the mineral density of calcaneous bone in postmenopausal women on hormonal therapy." *Journal of Reproductive Medicine,* vol. 35, no. 5, pp. 503–507, 1990.

12. Seelig MS, "Increased magnesium need with use of combined estrogen and calcium for osteoporosis." *Magnesium Res,* vol. 3, pp. 197–215, 1990.

13. Goldberg B, *Alternative Medicine Guide: Women's Health Series 2,* Future Medicine Publishing, Tiburon, CA, 1998.

14. Brown S, *Better Bones, Better Body,* Keats Publishing, New Canaan, CT, 1996.

15. Tucker KL et al., "Potassium, magnesium, and fruit and vegetable intakes are associated with greater bone mineral density in elderly men and women." *Am J Clin Nutr,* vol. 69, no. 4, pp. 727–736, 1999.

16. Hall WD et al., "Risk factors for kidney stones in older women in the southern United States." *Am J Med Sci,* vol. 322, no. 1, pp. 12–18, 2001.

17. Milne DB, Nielsen FH, "The interaction between dietary fructose

and magnesium adversely affects macromineral homeostasis in men." *J Am Coll Nutr,* vol. 19, no. 1, pp. 31–37, 2000.

18. Institute of Medicine. *Dietary Reference Intake for Calcium, Phosphorus, Magnesium, Vitamin D, and Fluoride,* National Academy Press, Washington DC, 1997.

19. Milne D, Nielsen F, "Too much soda may take some fizz out of the bones." *Proc ND Acad Sci,* vol. 51, p. 212, 1998.

20. Bunce GE et al., "Distribution of calcium and magnesium in rat kidney homogenate fractions accompanying magnesium deficiency induced nephrocalcinosis." *Exp Mol Pathol,* vol. 21, no. 1, pp. 16–28, 1974.

21. Johansson G et al., "Effects of magnesium hydroxide in renal stone disease." *J Am Coll Nutr,* vol. 1, no. 2, 1982.

22. Prien EL, "Magnesium oxide-pyridoxine therapy for recurring calcium oxalate urinary calculi." *J Urology,* vol. 112, pp. 509–551, 1974.

23. Johannson G et al., "Biochemical and clinical effects of prophylactic treatment of renal calcium stones with magnesium hydroxide." *J Urol,* vol. 124, pp. 770–774, 1980.

24. Driessens FC, Verbeeck RM, "On the prevention and treatment of calcification disorders of old age." *Med Hypotheses,* vol. 3, pp. 131–137, 1988.

25. Labeeuw M et al., "Role of magnesium in the physiopathology and treatment of calcium renal lithiasis." *Presse Med,* vol. 16, no. 1, pp. 25–27, 1987.

26. Massey L, "Magnesium therapy for nephrolithiasis." *Magnesium Research,*vol. 18, no. 12, pp. 123–126, 2005.

27. Jeppesen BB, "Greenland, a soft-water area with a low incidence of ischemic heart death." *Magnesium,* vol. 6, no. 6, pp. 307–313, 1987.

CHAPTER 12: CHRONIC FATIGUE SYNDROME AND FIBROMYALGIA

1. Goldstein JA, ed., *Chronic Fatigue Syndromes: The Limbic Hypothesis,* Haworth Press, New York, 1993.

2. Seelig MS, "Review and hypothesis: might patients with the chronic fatigue syndrome have latent tetany of magnesium deficiency." *J Chron Fatigue Syndr,* vol. 4, pp. 77–108, 1998.

3. Papadopol V, Tuchendria E, Palamaru I, "Magnesium and some psychological features in two groups of pupils (magnesium and psychic features)." *Magnes Research*, vol. 14, nos. 1–2, pp. 27–32, 2001.

4. Durlach V et al., "Neurotic, neuromuscular and autonomic nervous form of magnesium imbalance." *Magnes Res*, vol. 10, pp. 169–195, 1997.

5. Cox IM, "Red blood cell magnesium and chronic fatigue syndrome." *The Lancet*, vol. 337, pp. 757–760, 1991.

6. Goldberg B, *Chronic Fatigue, Fibromyalgia & Environmental Illness: 26 Doctors Show You How They Reverse These Conditions with Clinically Proven Alternative Therapies*, Future Medicine Publishing, Tiburon, CA, 1998.

7. Ibid.

8. Seelig MS, "Athletic stress, performance and magnesium in consequences of magnesium deficiency on the enhancement of stress reactions; preventive and therapeutic implications: a review." *J Am Coll Nutr*, vol. 13, no. 5, pp. 429–446, 1994.

9. Abraham GE, Flechas JD, "Management of fibromyalgia: rationale for the use of magnesium and malic acid." *P J Nutr Med*, vol. 3, pp. 49–59, 1992.

CHAPTER 13: ENVIRONMENTAL ILLNESS

1. "Nowhere to hide: persistent toxic chemicals in the U.S. food supply," Pesticide Action Network North America (PANNA) and Commonweal, 2000, available at http://www.panna.org/resources/documents/nowhereToHideAvail.dv.html.

2. "CDC releases most extensive assessment to date of Americans' exposure to environmental chemicals," Centers for Disease Control and Prevention telebriefing, January 31, 2003, www.cdc.gov/OD/OC/MEDIA/transcipts/t030131.htm.

3. "GAO finds that USDA, EPA have neglected pledge to cut pesticide use," U.S. General Accounting Office, U.S. Newswire, September 27, 2001, available at http://leahy.senate.gov/press/200109/010927.html.

4. Kreutzer R et al., "Prevalence of people reporting sensitivities to chemicals in a population-based survey." *Am J Epidemiol*, vol. 150, no. 1, pp. 1–12, 1999.

5. "Everyday carcinogens: stopping cancer before it starts." Workshop on Primary Cancer Prevention, McMaster University, Hamilton, Ontario, Canada, March 26–27, 1999.

6. Deborah Baker, personal communication. Dr. Baker shares her mercury research at www.y2khealthanddetox.com.

7. Goering PL et al., "Toxicity assessment of mercury vapor from dental amalgams." Fundam Appl Toxicol, vol. 19, no. 3, pp. 319–329, 1992.

8. Halbach S, "Amalgam tooth fillings and man's mercury burden. Review." Hum Exp Toxicol, vol. 13, no. 7, pp. 496–501, 1994.

9. Lorscheider FL et al., "Mercury exposure from 'silver' tooth fillings: emerging evidence questions a traditional dental paradigm." FASEB J, vol. 9, no. 7, pp. 504–508, 1995.

10. Arenholt-Bindslev D, Larsen AH, "Mercury levels and discharge in waste water from dental clinics." Water Air Soil Pollut, vol. 86, nos. 1–4, pp. 93–99, 1996.

11. Drasch G et al., "Comparison of the body burden of the population of Leipzig and Munich with the heavy metals cadmium, lead and mercury—a study of human organ samples." Gesundheitswesen, vol. 56, no. 5, pp. 263–267, 1994.

12. Liu XY, Jin TY, Nordberg GF, "Increased urinary calcium and magnesium excretion in rats injected with mercuric chloride." Pharmacol Toxicol, vol. 68, no. 4, pp. 254–259, 1991.

13. Durlach J, "Diverse applications of magnesium therapy, in Handbook of Metal-Ligand Interactions in Biological Fluids—Bioinorganic Medicine, vol. 2, Marcel Dekker, New York, 1995.

14. Kedryna T et al., "Effect of environmental fluorides on key biochemical processes in humans." Folia Med Cracov, vol. 34, no. 1–4, pp. 49–57, 1993.

15. Semczuk M, Semczuk-Sikora A, "New data on toxic metal intoxication (Cd, Pb, and Hg in particular) and Mg status during pregnancy. Review." Med Sci Monit, vol. 7, no. 2, pp. 332–340, 2001.

16. Ibid.

17. Durlach J et al., "Magnesium: a competitive inhibitor of lead and cadmium. Ultrastructure studies of the human amniotic epithelial cell." Magnesium Res, vol. 3, pp. 31–36, 1990.

18. Soldatovic D et al., "Contribution to interaction between magnesium and toxic metals: the effect of prolonged cadmium intoxication

on magnesium metabolism in rabbits." *Magnes Res,* vol. 11, no. 4, pp. 283–288, 1998.

19. Allen VG, "Influence of aluminum on magnesium metabolism," in Altura BM, Durlach J, Seelig MS, eds., *Magnesium in Cellular Processes and Medicine,* Krager, Basel, pp. 50–66, 1987.

20. Rogers S, *The EI Syndrome: A Rx for Environmental Illness.* Rev. ed. SK Publishing, Sarasota, FL, 1995.

CHAPTER 14: ASTHMA

1. Seelig M, "Consequences of magnesium deficiency on the enhancement of stress reactions; preventive and therapeutic implications (a review)." *J Am Coll Nutr,* vol. 13, no. 5, pp. 429–446, 1994.

2. *Physicians' Desk Reference,* 56th ed., Medical Economics, Oradell, NJ, 2002.

3. Gurkan F et al., "Intravenous magnesium sulphate in the management of moderate to severe acute asthmatic children nonresponding to conventional therapy." *Eur J Emerg Medicine,* vol. 6, no. 3, pp. 201–205, 1999.

4. Ciarallo L et al., "Intravenous magnesium therapy for moderate to severe pediatric asthma: results of a randomized, placebo-controlled trial." *J Pediatr,* vol. 129, pp. 809–814, 1996.

5. Dominguez LJ et al., "Bronchial reactivity and intracellular magnesium: a possible mechanism for the bronchodilating effects of magnesium in asthma." *Clin Sci (Colch),* vol. 95, no. 2, pp. 137–142, 1998.

6. Britton J, "Dietary magnesium, lung function, wheezing and airway hyperreactivity in a random population sample." *Lancet,* vol. 344, pp. 357–362, 1994.

CHAPTER 15: HEALTH AND LONGEVITY

1. Barbagallo M et al., "Cellular ionic alterations with age: relation to hypertension and diabetes." *J Am Geriatr Soc,* vol. 48, no. 9, pp. 1111–1116, 2000.

2. Barbagallo M, "Diabetes mellitus, hypertension and ageing: the ionic hypothesis of ageing and cardiovascular-metabolic diseases." *Diabetes Metab,* vol. 23, no. 4, pp. 281–294, 1997.

3. Hartwig A, "Role of magnesium in genomic stability." *Mutat Research,* vol. 18, no. 475 (1–2), pp. 113–121, 2001.

4. Worwag M et al., "Prevalence of magnesium and zinc deficiencies in nursing home residents in Germany." *Magnes Res*, vol. 12, no. 3, pp. 181–189, 1999.

5. Paolisso G et al., "Mean arterial blood pressure and serum levels of the molar ratio of insulin-like growth factor-1 to its binding protein-3 in centenarians." *J Hypertens*, vol. 17, pp. 67–73, 1999.

6. Li W et al., "Antioxidants prevent elevation in [Ca(2+)](i) induced by low extracellular magnesium in cultured canine cerebral vascular smooth muscle cells: possible relationship to Mg(2+) deficiency-induced vasospasm and stroke." *Brain Res Bull*, vol. 52, no. 2, pp. 151–154, 2000.

7. Hartwig A, "Role of magnesium in genomic stability." *Mutat Research*, vol. 18, no. 475 (1–2), pp. 113–121, 2001.

8. Blaylock RL, *Excitotoxins: The Taste That Kills*, Health Press, Sante Fe, NM, 1997.

9. Nelson L, "Pesticides and Parkinson's Disease," American Academy of Neurology 52nd Annual Meeting, San Diego, CA, April 29–May 6, 2000.

10. Blaylock RL, *Excitotoxins: The Taste That Kills*, Health Press, Sante Fe, NM, 1997.

11. Liu G, Slutsky I, "Magnesium may reverse middle-age memory loss." *MIT Tech Talk*, vol. 49, no. 12, December 8, 2004.

12. Rondeau V et al., "Aluminum in drinking water and cognitive decline in elderly subjects: the Paquid cohort." *Am J Epidemiol*, vol. 154, no. 3, pp. 288–290, 2001.

13. Rondeau V et al., "Relation between aluminum concentrations in drinking water and Alzheimer's disease: an 8-year follow-up study." *Am J Epidemiol*, vol. 152, pp. 59–66, 2000.

14. Andrasi E et al., "Disturbances of magnesium concentrations in various brain areas in Alzheimer's disease." *Magnes Res*, vol. 13, no. 3, pp. 189–196, 2000.

15. Yasui M et al., "Calcium, magnesium and aluminum concentrations in Parkinson's disease." *Neurotoxicology*, vol. 13, no. 3, pp. 593–600, 1992.

16. Blaylock RL, *Excitotoxins: The Taste That Kills*, Health Press, Sante Fe, NM, 1997.

17. Durlach J, "Diverse applications of magnesium therapy, in *Handbook*

of Metal-Ligand Interactions in Biological Fluids—Bioinorganic Medicine, vol. 2, Marcel Dekker, New York, 1995.

18. Blaylock RL, *Excitotoxins: The Taste That Kills,* Health Press, Sante Fe, NM, 1997.

19. Durlach J et al., "Magnesium and ageing. II. Clinical data: aetiological mechanisms and pathophysiological consequences of magnesium deficit in the elderly." *Magnes Res,* vol. 6, no. 4, pp. 379–394, 1993.

CHAPTER 16: MAGNESIUM REQUIREMENTS AND TESTING

1. Seelig MS, "The requirement of magnesium by the normal adult." *Am J Clin Nutr,* vol. 14, pp. 342–390, 1964.

2. Seelig MS, "Magnesium requirements in human nutrition." *Magnes Bull,* vol. 3 (1A), pp. 26–47, 1981.

3. Franz KB, "Magnesium intake during pregnancy." *Magnesium,* vol. 6, pp. 18–27, 1987.

4. Seelig MS, "The requirement of magnesium by the normal adult." *Am J Clin Nutr,* vol. 14, pp. 342–390, 1964.

5. Seelig MS, "Magnesium requirements in human nutrition." *Magnes Bull,* vol. 3 (1A), pp. 26–47, 1981.

6. Glei M et al., "Magnesium content of foodstuffs and beverages and magnesium intake of adults in Germany." *Magnes Bull,* vol. 17, pp. 22–28, 1995.

7. Cashman KD et al., "Optimal nutrition: calcium, magnesium, and phosphorous." *Proc Nutr Soc,* vol. 58, pp. 477–487, 1999.

8. Mircetic RN, Dodig S, Raos M, Petres B, Cepelak I, "Magnesium concentration in plasma, leukocytes and urine of children with intermittent asthma." *Clin Chim Acta,* vol. 312, nos. 1–2, pp. 197–203, 2001.

9. Ryzen E et al., "Parenteral magnesium tolerance testing in the evaluation of magnesium deficiency." *Magnesium,* vol. 4, pp. 137–147, 1985.

10. Burton Altura, personal communication, November 2001.

11. Altura BM, Altura BT, "Role of magnesium in patho-physiological processes and the clinical utility of magnesium ion selective electrodes." *Scand J Clin Lab Invest Suppl,* vol. 224, pp. 211–234, 1996.

12. Altura BT, Altura BM, "A method for distinguishing ionized, com-

plexed and protein-bound Mg in normal and diseased subjects." *Scand J Clin Lab Invest Suppl*, vol. 217, pp. 83–87, 1994.

13. Altura BT et al., "Comparative findings on serum IMg2+ of normal and diseased human subjects with the NOVA and KONE ISE's for Mg2+." *Scand J Clin Lab Invest Suppl*, vol. 217, pp. 77–81, 1994.

14. Altura BT et al., "Characterization of a new ion selective electrode for ionized magnesium in whole blood, plasma, serum, and aqueous samples." *Scand J Clin Lab Invest Suppl*, vol. 217, pp. 21–36, 1994.

15. Altura BT et al., "A new method for the rapid determination of ionized Mg2 in whole blood, serum and plasma." *Methods and Findings in Exp Clin Pharmacol*, vol. 4, pp. 297–304, 1992.

16. Altura BT, Altura BM, "Measurement of ionized magnesium in whole blood, plasma and serum with a new ion-selective electrode in healthy and diseased human subjects." *Magnes Trace Elem*, vol. 10, nos. 2–4, pp. 90–98, 1991–1992.

17. Altura BT, Altura BM, "A method for distinguishing ionized, complexed and protein-bound Mg in normal and diseased subjects." *Scand J Clin Lab Invest Suppl*, vol. 217, pp. 83–87, 1994.

18. Altura BM, Altura BT, "Role of magnesium in patho-physiological processes and the clinical utility of magnesium ion selective electrodes." *Scand J Clin Lab Invest Suppl*, vol. 224, pp. 211–234, 1996.

19. Ibid.

20. Personal communication with Burton Altura, November 2001.

21. Altura BT et al., "Clinical studies with the NOVA ISE for IMg2+." *Scand J Clin Lab Invest Suppl*, vol. 217, pp. 53–67, 1994.

22. Marcus JC, Altura BT, Altura BM, "Serum ionized magnesium in post-traumatic headaches." *J Pediatr*, vol. 139, no. 3, pp. 459–462, 2001.

23. Muneyvirci-Delale O et al., "Divalent cations in women with PCOS: implications for cardiovascular disease." *Gynecol Endocrinol*, vol. 3, pp. 198–201, 2001.

24. Marcus JC et al., "Serum ionized magnesium in premature and term infants." *Pediatr Neurol*, vol. 4, pp. 311–314, 1998.

25. Scott VL et al., "Ionized hypomagnesemia in patients undergoing orthotopic liver transplantation: a complication of citrate intoxication." *Liver Transpl Surg*, vol. 2, no. 5, pp. 343–347, 1996.

26. Altura BT et al., "Low levels of serum ionized magnesium are found

in patients early after stroke which result in rapid elevation in cytosolic free calcium and spasm in cerebral vascular muscle cells." *Neurosci Lett*, vol. 230, no. 1, pp. 37–40, 1997.

27. Handwerker SM, Altura BT, Altura BM, "Serum ionized magnesium and other electrolytes in the antenatal period of human pregnancy." *J Am Coll Nutr*, vol. 15, no. 1, pp. 36–43, 1996.

28. Memon ZI et al., "Predictive value of serum ionized but not total magnesium levels in head injuries." *Scand J Clin Lab Invest*, vol. 55, no. 8, pp. 671–677, 1995.

29. Handwerker SM, Altura BT, Altura BM, "Ionized serum magnesium and potassium levels in pregnant women with preeclampsia and eclampsia." *J Reprod Medicine*, vol. 40, no. 3, pp. 201–208, 1995.

CHAPTER 17: A MAGNESIUM EATING PLAN

1. Durlach J, Bac P, Bara M, Guiet-Bara A, "Cardiovasoprotective foods and nutrients: possible importance of magnesium intake." *Magnes Res*, vol. 12, no. 1, pp. 57–61, 1999.

2. Murray M, *Encyclopedia of Nutritional Supplements*, Prima Publishing, Rocklin, CA, 1996.

3. Wood M, *Seven Herbs: Plants as Teachers*, North Atlantic Books, Berkeley, CA, 1987.

4. Weed S, *Healing Wise: The Wise Woman Herbal*, Ash Tree Publishing, Woodstock, NY, 1989.

5. Duke JA, *The Green Pharmacy*, St. Martin's Press, New York, 1998.

6. Chevallier A, *The Encyclopedia of Medicinal Plants*, DK Publishing, New York, 1996.

7. Marx A et al., "Magnesium in drinking water and ischemic heart disease." *Epididemiol Rev*, vol. 19, pp. 258–272, 1997.

8. Von Wiesenberger A, *The Pocket Guide to Bottled Water*, Contemporary Books, Chicago, 1991.

CHAPTER 18: MAGNESIUM SUPPLEMENTATION AND HOMEOPATHIC MAGNESIUM

1. Durlach J, *Magnesium in Clinical Practice*, Libbey, London, 1988.

2. Fehlinger R, "Therapy with magnesium salts in neurological diseases." *Magnes Bull*, vol. 12, pp. 35–42, 1990.

3. Ducroix T, "L'enfant spasmophile—Aspects diagnostiques et théra-peutiques." *Magnes Bull,* vol. 1, pp. 9–15, 1984.

4. Seelig MS, "Athletic stress, performance and magnesium in con-sequences of magnesium deficiency on the enhancement of stress reactions; preventive and therapeutic implications: a review." *J Am Coll Nutr,* vol. 13, no. 5, pp. 429–446, 1994.

5. Chazov EI, Malchikova LS, Lipina NV, Asafov GB, Smirnov VN, "Tau-rine and electrical activity of the heart." *Circ Res,* vol. 35, suppl. 3, pp. 11–21, 1974.

6. Chahine R, Feng J, "Protective effects of taurine against reperfusion-induced arrhythmias in isolated ischemic rat heart." *Arzneimit-telforschung,* vol. 48, no. 4, pp. 360–364, 1998.

7. Seelig MS, "Magnesium requirements in human nutrition." *Magnes Bull,* vol. 3 (1A), pp. 26–47, 1981.

8. Johnson S, "The multifaceted and widespread pathology of magne-sium deficiency." *Med Hypotheses,* vol. 56, no. 2, pp. 163–170, 2001.

9. Rude RK et al., "Low serum concentrations of 1,25-dihydroxyvitamin D in human magnesium deficiency." *J Clin Endocrinol Metab,* vol. 61, pp. 833–940, 1985.

10. Fuss M et al., "Correction of low circulating levels of 1,25-dihydroxy-vitamin D by 25-hydroxyvitamin D during reversal of hypomagne-saemia." *Clinical Endocrinol Oxf,* vol. 31, pp. 31–38, 1989.

11. Manuel y Keenoy B, Moorkens G, Vertommen J, Noe M, Neve J, De Leeuw I, "Magnesium status and parameters of the oxidant-antioxidant balance in patients with chronic fatigue: effects of supplementation with magnesium." *J Am Coll Nutr,* vol. 19, no. 3, pp. 374–382, 2000.

12. Boericke OE, *Pocket Manual of Homeopathic Materia Medica,* 9th ed., Boericke & Runyon, Philadelphia, 1927.

INDEX

by, 203; anti-hypertensive,
9–10, 94–97, 101, 205;
asthma, 193; cholesterol,
88–89, 125; companies, 40,
56, 111; heart disease,
106–107, 110, 111–12;
interactions with
supplements in heart disease,
106–107; magnesium
deficiency and, 36–37, 175;
magnesium and prescription
drugs, 100; psychiatric, 45,
46, 55, 56–57
dry sauna, 188–89
dulse, 231
Durlach, Jean, 42, 206
dysmenorrhea (painful periods),
7, 11, 16, 138–39, 174

E
ear infections, 172
Eby, George, 224–25
eclampsia, 142
eczema, 173, 183, 191, 251
eggs, 237
electrical energy, 13–14, 75, 82
endometriosis, 11
energy, 13–14; low, 71;
producing and transporting,
14, 15
environmental illness, 180–90,
195, 200, 203, 204; diet
and, 187–88; metals,
185–86, 203; saunas for,
188–89; supplements for,
190; treatment, 182,
186–90
enzymes, 11, 12, 14, 15, 88, 90,
185, 200, 204; magnesium
and, 14, 15
epilepsy, 163
Epsom salts, 251
Epstein, Samuel, 184
Epstein-Barr virus, 167–68

Erasmus, Udo, 88
essential fatty acids, 90–91, 135,
137, 195, 227, 252–53
estrogen, 33, 63, 134–36, 179;
replacement, 152, 174
EXATest, 219–20
excitotoxins, 61
exercise, 6, 10, 58, 70–73, 153,
177; excessive, 71–73, 200;
lack of, 150; magnesium
and, 70–73
eyes: blurred vision, 93;
symptoms, in diabetics, 125,
126, 129; twitches, 45

F
far-infrared (FIR) sauna, 189
fast food, 11, 30, 35, 73, 85, 150
fasting, 188
fatigue, 45, 48, 171, 178–79,
207; chronic fatigue
syndrome, 167–71, 178–79
fats and oils, 23, 85–88, 116,
118, 200, 214, 224, 227,
237
fertilizers, 25–26
fever, 189
fiber, 85, 130, 214
fibromyalgia, 21, 157, 166,
170–77, 181, 246, 250;
diagnostic criteria, 170–71;
possible health chronology
for, 172–78; treatment, 179
fight-or-flight response, 49–50,
51, 52, 62
fish, 137, 227, 229, 237
fluid retention, 133, 134, 135
fluoride, 29, 38, 85
folic acid, 92, 150, 214
food, see diet; magnesium eating
plan; specific foods
food additives, 60–63, 74, 75,
176, 195
Ford, Robert, 87–88

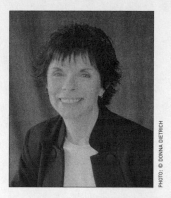

CAROLYN DEAN, M.D., N.D., has been in the forefront of health issues for twenty-eight years. She holds a medical license in California and is a graduate of the Ontario Naturopathic College and a former board member of the Canadian College of Naturopathic Medicine. Dr. Dean has authored and co-authored twelve books on the latest health issues of concern to the public. She is a consultant to Total Health for Longevity, First for Women, and Natural Health. She frequently has articles and interviews in various health magazines and appears on radio and television.

Dr. Carolyn Dean is both a medical doctor and naturopathic doctor who assists individuals with all types of illness at any stage or degree of severity. Dr. Dean specializes in managing and healing often misdiagnosed and chronic conditions, such as digestive problems, hormone imbalance, recurring infection, irritable bowel syndrome, widespread inflammation, allergies, anxiety, fibromyalgia, mood swings, chronic fatigue syndrome, fluid retention, lost vitality, and many other conditions that often remain unresolved. For most patients, Dr. Dean assists in halting disease progression and preventing symptoms from worsening. Feeling better and regaining a former state of better health are attainable goals in many cases. Dr. Dean offers private, customized Consultations for Health by phone. You can reach Dr. Dean at www.carolyndean.com.